It's All About The Work!

It's All About The Work!

*My Recovery from a Stroke
And Discovery of a New Normal*

By G. Ross Kelly

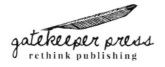

gatekeeper press
rethink publishing

It's All About The Work!
My Recovery from a Stroke
And Discovery of a New Normal

Published by Gatekeeper Press
3971 Hoover Rd. Suite 77
Columbus, OH 43123-2839

ISBN (hardcover): 9781619846937
ISBN (paperback): 9781619846944

Printed in the United States of America

With excerpts from....

Steve Burrell

Yolanda Giddens

and

Frederick Blair

Edited by

Jennifer Parker

Dedication

Some will say this book is merely an effort to applaud the nursing community.... it is.

Some will say it is intended to do the same for physical, speech and occupational therapists.... it is.

Some will say it is an opportunity to honor my large, close-knit family.... it is.

Or perhaps some will say it is about the friends, caretakers and support groups that have provided their love and support through this ordeal....   it is.

And many are convinced it is an attempt to celebrate the community of stroke survivors and caregivers and their journeys to regain their dignity and normalcy.... it is.

It is about all of those things and more. This book is dedicated to those who have endured such an ordeal, and the group of professionals, family and friends that were instrumental in my recovery... their professionalism, their expertise, and most of all, their hearts. It is because of them that this book was written and because of them it was able to be written.

Table of Contents

Introduction

A Good Life
Temporarily Interrupted

MINE HAS BEEN A GOOD LIFE. I enjoyed a 30+ year career in the consulting industry with companies including Digital Equipment Corporation, Compaq Computer and Hewlett Packard, and had embarked on a second career as a writer and songwriter. I had written and published the story of my family, and was engaged in a series of ghost writing projects with other aspiring authors. Additionally, I was conducting workshops for those who wished to write their story.

I had three grown children and eight grandchildren who I adored and was enjoying watching them grow to become wonderful and responsible adults. I had a former wife and, though divorced, we maintained a close and loving relationship. We remained good parents after our divorce and were now good grandparents together, as well as good friends. I had a woman in my life who I was devoted to.

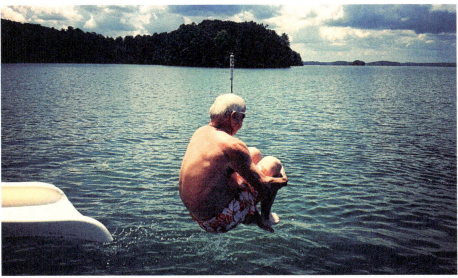

Living life

I maintained a healthy lifestyle. I exercised every day. I ate healthy. My friends ridiculed me for my diet. Every morning I made a fruit smoothie and during the day would do my best to avoid glutens and other foods that are deemed harmful or fat producing. My cholesterol and blood pressure were normal. I did not smoke or have diabetes. I maintained my weight. I showed no indication or predictive behaviors as to what was to come.

My life could have been characterized by the Joe Walsh song, "*Life's been good to me so far.*"

I have a wonderful family. I enjoyed an exceptional career. I was now doing what I enjoyed most, my writing and my music. I enjoyed good health. I was a former marathoner. I traveled the world from Rio to Tokyo and every country in between, and had enjoyed many professional and leisurely activities.

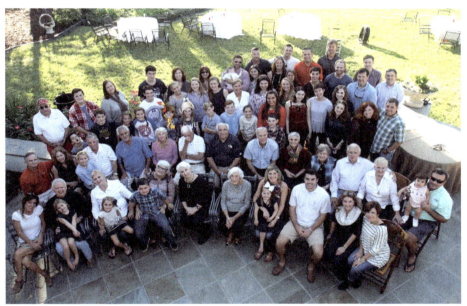

A typical Kelly Thanksgiving

That is until one morning I woke up and my body began to vibrate like I had stuck my finger in a light socket. I was rarely sick and certainly not accustomed to being dependent on others for my basic survival needs, but that's where I found myself.

How do you go from being a healthy human being one minute to become a virtual invalid the next? I suppose a fall could do the trick, or a car crash, or some other malady. I found myself in that condition by virtue of a stroke.

I was told I did not exactly fit the profile of a typical stroke victim... with one minor exception... my father had died of a stroke at the age of 70.

When they asked me in the hospital about family history, I robotically responded no family history to indicate stroke until they asked me if my father was still alive. I responded, "No, he died of a stroke at age 70." As the words came out of my mouth, the realization hit me...

He died of a stroke at age 70... Family history.

THE WORDS ECHOED IN MY head the same way my body had vibrated at the time of my stroke. Is *that* the reason I'm here?

I suddenly found myself in a new place, a new world. But there was no time to ruminate. It had not fully hit me at the time, but I was trying to absorb the fact that my life had taken a drastic change. Instead of being the one who would show regard and care for others when they were sick, I was now that one. At the time, there was too much going on for me to fully realize what had happened.

I landed in the emergency room of what was regarded as one of the finest medical facilities in the country, undergoing a triage procedure that consisted of a series of tests and procedures to determine the severity of my condition, and what would be needed to get me stabilized and on the road to recovery.

I was told that on a scale of 100, my stroke was on the lighter side in the lower teens. I found that interesting because my right leg and right arm and hand were completely paralyzed. I wondered what a more severe stroke might consist of. I had lost no cognitive abilities that I was aware of.

After I was stabilized and the emergency room crew had completed their work, I was transferred to the critical care section of the hospital to monitor my condition over the next two or three days, which I was told was standard protocol. It was only after my second day in the hospital that my new reality began to sink in. I had suffered a stroke. The shock and denial slowly gave way to that realization. My life as an entertainer, a writer, an athlete, a workshop facilitator, a man of leisure, a man of control and cool, had all come to an abrupt end.

Or had it?

IT WAS TOO EARLY IN the process to know what was in store for me. My initial thought was, "OK, a couple of days in the hospital and, boom, I go home and things return to normal." I even made that comment to a couple of nurses. Though they didn't comment out loud, but I'm sure they thought to themselves "Yeah, right. He doesn't have a clue." They were right. I didn't have a clue.

I had still not informed my family. My naïve belief was, this will pass and once I get back home I will let them know what had happened. So, until then, nothing to see here. It was just a temporary blip, and all is better now. Everything is back to normal. Ha!

I slowly came to the conclusion that would not be the case. I was somewhat out of the woods, and no longer in a fight for my survival, but I was in for a long recovery period that would require a great deal of work on my part. The realization was beginning to sink in. My initial reactions of anger and denial had begrudgingly become acceptance and determination. I began to re-frame the situation in my mind… "Okay, I've had tough battles in my life and was able to overcome them. This would be one of those."

I didn't know what the nature of that battle would be, but I began to prepare for a fight. I thought to myself, "How would an overweight person go about a commitment to lose 100 pounds?" It becomes a job… like going to the gym every day.

This would now be my job.

After eventually letting my children and the rest of my family know what had happened, they immediately mobilized to determine what would be needed as I embarked on the road to my recovery. While I was in the hospital, my family, and especially my children, along with Jennifer and Brenda, my former wife, took on the job of planning and helping me manage the communication of what had happened. The nursing staff would have the burden of doing the heavy lifting and acting as my primary caregivers. The family's work as caregivers would commence once I left the hospital and was back home. None of us knew fully what to expect at the time, but the reality of the situation was taking shape.

My oldest son, Brett, lived in Maryland, some 600 miles away. He came down on multiple occasions to be a part of my recovery, and when he was not physically here, he continued to be present through texts, phone and emails every day. It felt like he was next-door.

The same can be said of my second son, Rob. He lived in Chattanooga, but managed to make the three hour drive to the hospital weekly, if not two or three times a week. He, his wife Jill, and their three daughters made their presence in my life felt weekly, if not daily.

Erin, the youngest of my three children, was my only daughter and lived close by. She was close enough to be in and out of the hospital on a daily basis, and served as my head cheerleader. In addition to being daddy's little girl, she was a fitness coach herself, and had become an active member of my recovery team. In the end, she became my toughest coach.

It was clear to me, both through their presence and their actions, that I had three take-charge adult children now looking after my interests.

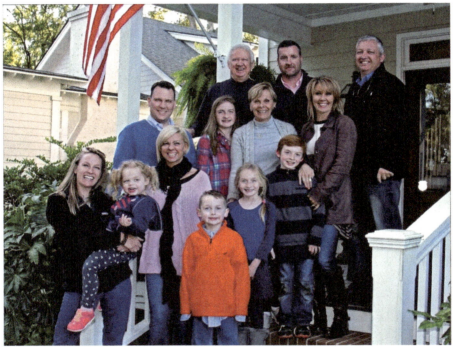

My immediate family.
Front row: Erin Kelly Knight, Grace Kelly, Finnegan Kelly.
Second row: Patti Kelly, Juliet Knight.
Third row: Brett Kelly, Isabel Knight, Brenda Kelly, Grayson Knight, Jill Kelly.
Top row: Me, Randy Knight, Rob Kelly.

Thankfully, this is the first time my children had to mobilize in this fashion, and when the bell rang, they answered the call. At the time, I was too oblivious to appreciate all they were doing behind the curtains, but before my eyes, my three children were now the grown-ups in charge. And I could not be more proud and thankful.

As the days progressed, I continued to receive praise, both by the hospital staff and my family, for my attitude and how hard I was working. They continued to express how encouraged they were by my determination to fight. I, in contrast, was impatient and eager to see more progress. Improvements began to occur but they seemed to come painfully and slowly. I continually asked the medical staff how long this would take, and was continually given the same answer, "It depends. Every situation is different." While I knew in my heart that was the case, the answer nonetheless was frustrating.

Gradually, I began to formulate my own answer. Whether my recovery was going to take 1000 steps or 15,000 steps, I determined that each step would have to be navigated, one by one, and no steps could be bypassed. There were no shortcuts. Concluding that to be the case, I gradually began to think less about how long or how many steps it would take, and more about simply embarking on the steps, one at a time. I had to accept what had happened to me, but not allow myself to be defined by it.

That conclusion changed my attitude and approach to my recovery and therapy. No longer would the sessions be an intrusion into asking my body to do things when it would not or could not perform. They would serve as my road to recovery. It would be my therapy sessions that would enable me to navigate each and every one of those steps, whether 1000 or 15,000.

I still continued to ask how long it would take, but I knew the answer.

My life, both in the hospital and when I returned home from the hospital, had become simply a matter of doing the work. If I was asked to do 25 repetitions of a particular exercise, I would do 30. What if I did 50? Would that help me navigate those steps faster? While the hospital staff and family applauded my effort, I was continually reminded to devote periods of time to rest to allow my body do what bodies need to do to heal. I failed miserably at that task. For me, every moment was an opportunity to exercise, even when I was in my bed, supposedly asleep. There were many nights, sometimes at 3 AM, I found myself moving or attempting to move certain parts of my body that had yet to reawaken.

After four weeks in the hospital, I was discharged to go home and continue my therapy on an outpatient basis. Little did I know or appreciate the journey I had embarked upon. It would be longer than I thought. It would be more frustrating than I thought. It would be tougher than I thought. But I eventually began to see a flicker of light at the end of the tunnel.

This is the story of that journey. How I recovered, and how I found my new normal.

CHAPTER 1
That Morning

Day One

THIS WAS THE YEAR I was going to surprise everyone. This was the year I was going to take care of my Christmas shopping before the actual holiday. My children were now adults and my focus on my grandchildren was more about their college fund than gifts. And my family members had grown beyond gift giving. But, there was still work to be done and I was determined to do it. My plan was to devote the early part of the week to some serious shopping even though most of it would be done online.

It was the Monday before the Christmas weekend. I woke up and made coffee, as I do every morning. I got back in bed with my morning coffee to catch up on the news, sports, Facebook and other daily check-in's, as I do every morning. I finished my coffee and got up to make a fruit smoothie, as I do every morning. When I stood up, however, my entire body began to vibrate. I didn't know what it was but I knew something was wrong. I reached for the wall. It was visible to me, but blurry. I could not reach it. I stumbled.

Jennifer, my girlfriend, lived 45 minutes away but her work was closer to my house, and occasionally she would stay with me. She was on the verge of retirement but was still working three days a week. Fortunately, she had stayed over with me the night before. She was in the other side of the house preparing for a routine Monday at work.

I called out to her, but being in another part of the house behind closed doors, she could not hear me. I waited for what seemed like an eternity for her to come out to the living area. When she did and was finally in ear shot of me, I told her I had stumbled and was unable to walk. Just as with members of my family, I had joked with her once too often and she wondered if I was joking now. She quickly realized by the expression on my face that I was not.

Once she understood the seriousness of the situation, she quickly came to my aide. After I told her the sensations I was feeling, she immediately concluded I was having a stroke. She is a nurse practitioner and thankfully knew the symptoms.

She asked if I wanted her to call 911. Anticipating the commotion it would cause in my neighborhood, and the length of time it would take for them to arrive, I told her no. That being said, she told me to get in her car because she was driving me to the hospital. No questions asked.

That was a life-saving moment.

She not only knew enough to recognize I was having a stroke, but also acted quickly and decisively at a time when I was unable to do so on my own. Her actions clearly saved my life.

The next thing I knew I was in the emergency room of the Northeast Georgia Medical Center.

What took place next was all a blur to me. All I knew was that I was in one of the leading hospitals in the country for strokes and heart related issues. Jennifer later told me the ER doctors had executed a triage protocol consisting of a series of tests that the hospital routinely performs in the event of a suspected stroke. Knowing her way around a hospital setting, she seemed sufficiently impressed with the way the emergency room staff went about their business.

At the conclusion of the tests and diagnosis, I was transferred to the critical care unit in the hospital. I was still groggy from the morning's fast moving events, and thankfully Jennifer was more in tune than I. She was not only more aware of what was happening and more knowledgeable, she had taken notes...

From Jennifer's notes...

December 19

About 7:45 a.m, got out of bed, R leg and arm were limp.

Fell down C/o dizziness.

On the way to hospital. N & V (nausea and vomiting)

To ER by 8:27am

Tests @ 8:35 (CT)

TPA (clot buster) given 8:58am (has to be given within 4 hr)

Stroke scale of 1-100, went from 2 to 11 and is stable.

11:15-2nd CT scan. First one was clear. No bleeding. Ischemic stroke.

2nd CT was clear but due to contrast from the1st one, want to make sure there was nothing obscuring the test.

12:15pm to ICU

Lupa is speech therapist, Meagan nurse

David...heart "bubble test" @ 2:15

MRI @ 8:48pm

December 20th

Jenny-OT @ 8:15am.

Lynn and Britney-PT @ 9:30

Neurology Añn Marie (Dr. Paquaio)-Small vessel stroke in the pons. Rehab, BP and cholesterol meds with 325 ASA daily.

Moved to room 1132 this evening

December 21st

Slept well. Ate well at breakfast. Had Asa, blood thinner injection and stool softener. Neurologist says he will prescribe Lisinopril for BP.

9:15am- PT walked in hall

Ashley is Tech. Her parents are coming for Christmas. Got Ross up to BS toilet.

Had Speech therapy and OT.

Sat up most of day, back in bed @ 6:30 pm

Funny note… Ross's face was red and all the staff was worried that he was overworking; turns out he used shower gel for what he thought was after shave and left it on. Had an allergic reaction and accidentally exfoliated his whole face.

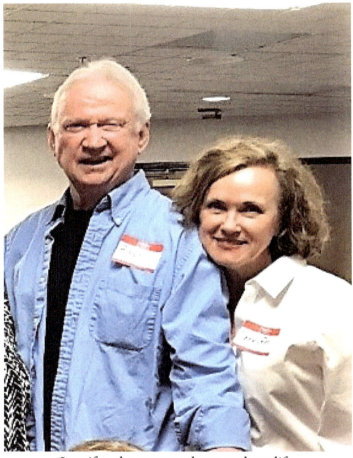
Jennifer, the woman that saved my life.

Tests revealed my stroke had not caused bleeding to my brain, which was a good thing. Mine was described as an ischemic stroke, one which occurs as a result of a clot in a one of the blood vessels supplying blood to the brain. If they had discovered bleeding in the brain, it would have been characterized as a hemorrhagic stroke, which is when a weakened blood vessel ruptures, and causes the bleeding. That would have been more serious. Hemorrhagic strokes account for only about 15% of all strokes, and fortunately, mine was not one. Having determined that mine was ischemic, no bleeding, that allowed them to administer what is referred to as a clot busting drug designed to dissolve the blood clot that created the obstruction.

I was also told, based on the test they administered, my stroke was on the lower end of the scale in terms of severity. I had no frame of reference for what a stroke on the lower end of the scale is supposed to feel like, but I was surprised by that assessment, as I was completely unable to move my right leg and right arm and hand. That paralysis, I was told, is referred to as a hemiparesis, a paralysis on one side of the body. If mine was relatively minor, I remember wondering what a more severe stroke must feel like.

My first few hours in critical care were also a blur to me. I just remember nurses checking in on me what seemed like every five minutes, and continuously monitoring my vital signs.

I gradually began to regain my senses enough to engage the nurses and medical staff and learn that I was the newest member of a growing fraternity of stroke survivors. It was a fraternity not of my choosing. The reality of my situation was becoming clearer.

One of the critical care nurses was named Bradee (Yes, that's how she spells her name. Take it up with her parents). She was a tall attractive woman, and as it turned out, her mother was the president and CEO of the hospital. Also, ironically, she told me that her father had recently suffered a stroke and was in the hospital, enduring an experience similar to mine. She was determined that I meet him.

I was very appreciative of the connection. Steve Burrell would be the first fellow member to welcome me into my new fraternity and would become the first of a group of new lifelong friends that I would cultivate from this experience. I was not happy about how we became friends, but was thankful for the friendship. He was about a week ahead of me in his recovery and would serve as a guide to educate me on what was ahead of me. I would later learn more about his experience, which is shared in this book.

Day 4

THIS WAS NOT THE CHRISTMAS week I had in mind. As much of the world was going about their business preparing for the holiday season, I was busy trying to get my right thumb to move. My mind said 'move', but my body refused to respond. Is *this* what the next 3 to 6 months of my life was going to be … working to regain the use of one body part at a time? The right side of my body was still paralyzed, and the severity of that paralysis was just becoming clear to me. It was going to be a long road.

After two days in intensive care, I was deemed to be out of immediate danger and was transferred to a general unit in the hospital. The new location did not provide the same level of personalized care as I had experienced in the ICU, but the treatment and accommodations were still very good.

As I watched the nurses go through their routines, I found myself reverting to my old consulting practice. I began to analyze the procedures being carried out to attempt to assess the quality of the care that was provided. Vital sign checks, for example, were extended from every five minutes to every hour. Medication was administered on a regular basis. I was readjusted in my bed every hour, whether it was needed or not. There seemed to be a purpose for everything. They had strict protocols. It was very impressive. Hopefully, it would all lead to a happy conclusion.

After two days in my new room, I was visited by a member of the therapeutic staff who told me I may qualify to undergo rehab in the hospital. I didn't know what tests I would have to take to determine my qualification, but a rehabilitation unit seemed like the place I would want to go if I were going to get this thing behind me. I hoped the assessment would not require physical activities of any sort, as I remained paralyzed. It turned out to be simply a routine assessment of my condition and circumstances. I was soon told that I qualified. Move number three.

The transfer was rather painless. I quickly found myself in surroundings that seemed less like a hospital and more like a live-in gymnasium. I was now in the therapeutic or rehab unit of the hospital. Here, I was told, I would undergo a regimen of speech, occupational and physical therapies to help me begin my road to recovery. At the time, I didn't know the difference between the three types of therapies. I only knew that I would be up in the morning, take my breakfast as well as other meals out in a general cafeteria setting with the other patients, and then head off to work. It was clear that I was in a different setting, and one that would involve work. I did not yet know the nature or the extensiveness of the work, but it was clear that work would be the centerpiece of my stay.

Unfortunately my therapies got off to a shaky start. At some point during my hospital stay, I contracted a virus of some sort, causing vomiting and diarrhea. As a result, I missed my first day of work. Being paralyzed AND nauseous at the same time was not a pleasant combination, but I reminded myself that there are many in this hospital that experience something like that every day. My circumstance, I concluded, was merely one of temporary inconvenience. There were others who didn't have that luxury.

After 24 hours of sickness, I was finally deemed healthy enough to proceed. I soon found myself in the gym being asked to execute a series of tasks that my body simply would not or could not perform. I was unable to even sit up without support. Now, I was really beginning to understand the extent of my paralysis.

Day 6

THE HOLIDAY SEASON WOULD BE proceeding without me this year. The gifts I had ordered had not yet been picked up and I missed the traditional family holiday party being hosted by my niece, Emily, and her husband, Nic. Even the medical staff at the hospital seemed to be going about their business as if it were just another workday. There was little mention that this was Christmas morning.

The holiday festivities eventually began when my family arrived later in the afternoon. I was deluged with a collection of gifts, cards and other offerings to celebrate the holiday. I was already emotional as a result of what had happened to me, and the celebration made me even more so. I had been told that a stroke has the tendency to heighten your emotions. I now fully felt it. As the family sat around my bed celebrating the holiday, I cried like a newborn baby. It was only then that I began to fully feel the emotions of what had happened to me and the life I would be living for the foreseeable future.

When I was not in the gym working, I was in my bed or sitting in my wheelchair in my room. During those times, if I did not have visitors, ESPN had become my primary companion. It was the holiday football bowl season, and trapped in my bed with nowhere to go, I found myself watching games between schools I barely knew. In between the regular check-in's by the nurses, my therapy sessions, and the visits from Jennifer and my family, I was glued to the TV. Who else was interested in the Armed Forces Bowl, or the Dollar General Bowl or the Hawaii or St. Pete Bowls, other than maybe those who had attended the schools, or their family members? The answer was the 173 people in the stands and me. If nothing else, I was learning about holiday bowl games I never knew existed.

The big game I was waiting for was the national championship game between Clemson and Alabama. Monikka, one of the nurses on the unit, was an avid Clemson Tigers fan, and she shared my anticipation for that one. The game would not only be the highlight of the bowl season, but also would be a celebration of Deshaun Watson, the local high school football star who was now the quarterback for the Clemson team and one of the top college recruits in the nation. Meanwhile, we were entertained with a steady diet of games such as the Cactus, Pinstripe, Russell Athletic and Foster Farms bowls, among many others.

Without looking, quick: where is the TaxSlayer bowl?

Beyond my newfound courtship with ESPN and the nonstop series of college bowl games, I was getting acclimated to my new surroundings. The nurses were good, my room was comfortable and the care was excellent. If you're going to have to have a stroke, I thought to myself, this was not a bad way to recover, even if I still couldn't move the right side of my body.

I was living a kind of schizophrenic life... by day, I was a workout freak, even if my body refused to cooperate, and in between sessions, I was lying in my bed like a couch potato, vegging on football.

Day 13

NEW YEAR'S DAY ARRIVED WITHOUT fanfare. Other than the occasional 'Happy New Year' being heard in adjacent rooms or in the hallway, January 1 could have been any other day of the year. Later in the day, I enjoyed visits from Jennifer and family members to celebrate the holiday and remind me that 2017 had finally arrived. Throughout the celebrations, I thought to myself how I was looking forward to the new year, especially given the way the previous year had ended.

Though I knew they were essential to my recovery, the first few therapy sessions had not been fun. I was failing at everything I was being asked to do. When asked to stand on my own, my legs refused. When asked to raise my right arm, it barely trembled. Walking was out of the question, even with assistance, as was picking up anything with my right hand. I was able to speak in coherent sentences during my speech therapy sessions, but otherwise, I was a complete flop. There I was, a healthy human being and former marathon runner, unable to stand, walk, or execute the most routine tasks. Meanwhile, I could not help but notice others around me in the gym who were working on similar tasks and the progress they were making and wonder to myself if I would ever be at that level.

My self-imposed three month timeline was beginning to feel more like six.

My therapy sessions had become a series of exercises in being asked to do something my body was not yet prepared to do. For the first few days, I dreaded the process. I was not only failing but the exercises were exhausting. My body had been assaulted and I was just beginning to realize how badly.

After a few sessions, however, I began to think… Therapy was the only way I would regain my sense of normalcy. Therapy was the only way I would walk naturally again... talk naturally again... or raise my arm above my head. I concluded every one there understood what had happened to me and did not judge me for my inability to perform. They were there to help. I gradually began to view my therapy differently. It would be my pathway back to normalcy. Looking back, I now understand those initial failures on my part were not a pass or fail, but merely a very humbling baseline from which to begin my journey. This was my starting point. Things would only get better, eventually.

With the college bowl season and holidays behind me, and 2017 awaiting, my new journey was underway. I had work to do.

CHAPTER 2
Doctors, Nurses and Therapists, Oh My

I HAD BEEN HOSPITALIZED ONCE before, years ago, but did not remember or appreciate the role nurses played in my recovery. This time I did. Perhaps it was because, this time, I was a virtual invalid and dependent on nurses for practically everything. I had lost total movement on the right side of my body, which means I could not walk, I could not feed myself, I could not go to the bathroom, take a shower, or even get dressed without assistance. I had to depend on someone else for my every move. Without fail, the nurses thankfully were there to provide that assistance.... and they did so graciously and willingly. I was struck by how helping another seemed to come so naturally to them.

That was even more true for the nurse's aides or nurse technicians. Before my stroke, my morning regimen was accomplished without thought or effort. I could now no longer perform the basic routine tasks of preparing for my day. That is where the nurses and nurse technicians stepped in. They were not only accustomed to helping us do what we could not do on our own, they did so without question. That was their job. And they performed it without hesitation.

My morning typically began with a nurse technician waking me and preparing me for breakfast. That also meant transferring me from the bed to a wheelchair, which was my only source of mobility. Once in the wheelchair and somewhat presentable, I would navigate my way to the breakfast area to join the other patients, using my left foot and left hand to power and guide myself. Occasionally, I took breakfast in my room. Either way, it was not without the assistance of one of the nurse technicians.

Ever try buttering a piece of toast or opening a package of jelly without the use of one hand?

Also, my morning regimen consisted of one of the nurses administering a newly prescribed cocktail of my daily medications and taking my vital signs. Most of my medications were taken orally, but one was administered by a daily injection in the stomach. The bruises on my stomach from the injections served as a stark reminder that I was indeed in a different world.

After breakfast, I clumsily managed my way through the process of brushing my teeth, combing my hair, and getting ready for my morning therapy session. In those earliest days, it was a nurse technician who performed the basic functions of helping me dress, and tie my shoes. I was capable of doing very little for myself, and when I did, it was agonizingly slow and exhausting. Fortunately, no request for assistance was out of bounds for the nursing staff. I was not accustomed to requiring assistance to put on my shoes or change my underwear. They earned their paychecks.

At times, I was uncomfortable and somewhat embarrassed about having to rely on the nurses and nurse technicians to assist me with my most fundamental tasks. I wanted to do things for myself. I wanted to prove, to them and me, that I had limitations but could still do things on my own. I quickly learned to overlook that issue. They were neither uncomfortable nor embarrassed with whatever task that needed to be performed, and they did so with a smile on their face. Vanity and modesty were not their concern, only wellness and recovery.

As the days passed, I was getting to know as much about the nursing staff as they knew about me. I thought how they had their own lives to live, families to take care of, mortgages to pay, sick babies to tend to, and all the other matters of living. Yet, they somehow managed to leave those issues at home, and devote their time in the hospital to the patients in their care. I was not surprised by the many issues in their own lives, but was pleasantly surprised by their ability to compartmentalize and focus on the task at hand.

From my brief stay with Bradee and the other nurses in the ICU, to my more extended stay with nurses in the therapy unit, Jennifer, the three Crystals, Monikka, Taye, and the many others saw me through my darkest days. The nurses and nurse technicians had become my Angels of Mercy at a time when I was more dependent than at any time in my life.

Many nights when I was awake doing exercises at 3 AM instead of sleeping, and they came in to perform their hourly bed checks and check my vital signs, those routine checks turned into enjoyable, personable conversations. They were now an extension of my family, and would be the first of my many caregivers throughout my recovery.

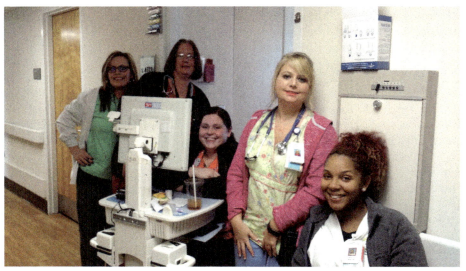

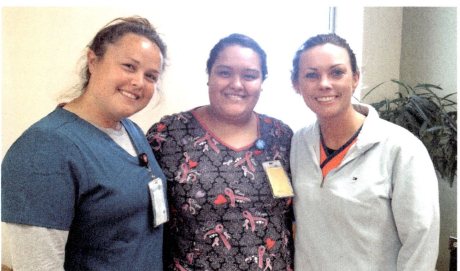

Just a few of the many angels.
Top picture, L to R:Sharon Coley, Janet Howard,Brittany Deal,
Crystal Doolittle and Taye Jones.
Bottom picture, L to R, Lauren Gillespie, Lucy Mata and Crystal Leach.

One aspect of my hospital stay that I had not anticipated was being fully
alarmed everywhere I went. My bed was alarmed to notify the nursing staff

if I made any attempt to get out of bed. My wheelchair, which was my only mode of transportation, was also alarmed. It was if I had been viewed as some sort of flight risk and they were determined to know my whereabouts at all times. I felt like a prisoner being monitored with an ankle bracelet. I was reminded that the real reason for this precaution was to prevent me from doing anything foolish or harmful to myself, such as attempting to get out of bed or out of my wheelchair. Falling was against the rules in the hospital, and the nursing staff was determined that I abided by that rule.

The irony was during the early days of my stay, I didn't have the strength or capability to get out of bed or out of my wheelchair on my own because the entire right side of my body was useless. But as the days progressed and my body began to regain some of its movement, the alarms had become a necessary precaution. In the spirit of true confession, I must admit that on more than one occasion, I was guilty of attempting to stand or get out of bed at a time when I was most likely a risk to myself. Each time, the intercom would blare, "Mr. Kelly, please remain in your bed." Big Sister was listening.

I was beginning to appreciate much about the nurses, nurse technicians, and the nursing profession during my stay at the hospital. They may not have been completely responsible for my recovery, but they were certainly essential to my well-being at a time when I was vulnerable and unable to perform the basic functions of getting out of bed and preparing for my day. I developed a new appreciation for the nursing staff and the role they played in sustaining me through the most difficult time of my life. And though I know differently, they always made me feel as if I was the only patient in the unit. Like teachers, I concluded, they were underpaid and underappreciated for all that they do.

The therapists were no different. If the role of nurses and nurse technicians was to ensure that I was able to sustain myself as I embarked on my recovery, the role of the therapists was to show me the way.

When I was transferred to the therapy unit and had overcome my brief sickness, I was there to begin my long and rocky road back to normalcy. The first thing I learned was the different roles the therapists played. Speech therapy, as I defined it, was from the throat up, and focused on cognitive issues, language issues, the ability to speak clearly, chewing and swallowing, and the many other things related to the face and throat that we take for granted. Occupational therapy was from the shoulders down and focused on the ability to perform the most routine tasks such as dressing myself and taking a shower, as well as the many other daily activities of living. Physical therapy, which would be the most strenuous of my sessions, focused on my ability to stand and walk. That would be my biggest challenge.

Once I understood the different roles and after initially viewing them as an intrusion, I began to appreciate their jobs and the role each would play in my recovery.

In those early days, my speech resembled a drunk at a bar at 2:30 in the morning telling a story of past exploits, whether you wanted to hear it or not. Additionally, the right side of my face was completely shut down. It was the task of Jen Zonts, an attractive and caring, but matter-of-fact speech therapist, to guide me through the process of correcting that. I did not envy her task.

She was instrumental in the recovery of my speech and facial expression, but, over time, she became so much more. She also became my attitude coach. Regaining my speech was a matter of facial exercises and repetitions of speaking more clearly, which meant practicing conversations that used difficult words to test the quality of speech. Jen was the queen of tongue twisters. We not only used difficult words and phrases to test and recover my speech, but spoke about subjects that would make our conversations more personally relevant to my life and hers.

I felt some of the drills would be difficult for anyone, much less someone recovering from a stroke. Try saying the word 'sorority' or 'colloquialism' five times real fast, with clarity.

I know. I couldn't do it either.

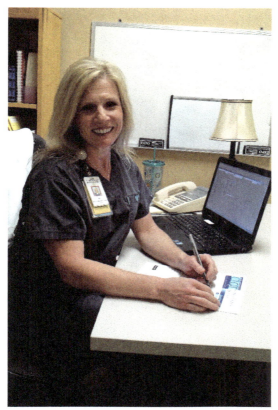

Jen Zonts, my speech therapist and attitude coach.

My occupational therapists were two, equally attractive, caring and dedicated women named Niki Redstrom and Charlie Chapman (Not to be confused with *Charlie Chaplin*). Their focus was helping me regain my ability to perform day-to-day tasks for myself around the home and community. They had the unenviable challenge of helping me regain my independence. From getting dressed, to showering, to cooking, to driving, I had to re-learn how to live as an independent human being. That task fell to them, and again I was beginning from a point of failure. Whether erasing a chalkboard or moving objects from one bucket to another, the most fundamental exercise they posed was overwhelming.

Those early days seemed like a rugged, mountainous road and they had to continuously convince me that progress would eventually come. I had no choice but to take them at their word. Like Jen, they showed as much concern for my emotional well-being as they did my physical recovery.

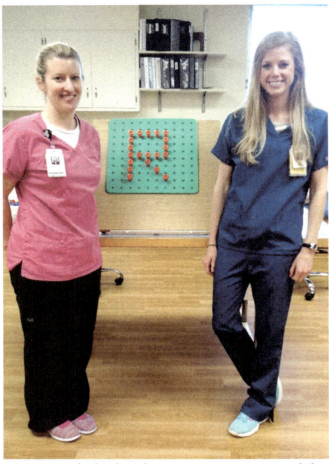

Niki Redstrom and Charlie Chapman, my occupational therapists.

My physical therapy was focused on helping me relearn how to stand and walk comfortably and without a limp. That was the most grueling and visible aspect of my condition, and was led by a big, bearish, teddy bear of a man, named Gray Riggsbee.

When I was practicing conversations during my speech therapy with Jen, I was not visible to others. The same was basically true when I was moving marbles or other objects with my hands during occupational therapy with Niki and Charlie. But everyone in the gymnasium was able to watch as I wobbled in my attempts to stand and walk. My failures were there for the world to see.

Gray, a jovial but determined man, made my exercises challenging. I was eager to recover and wanted to be pushed, and he didn't hesitate to push me. My body was just not ready to fully cooperate.

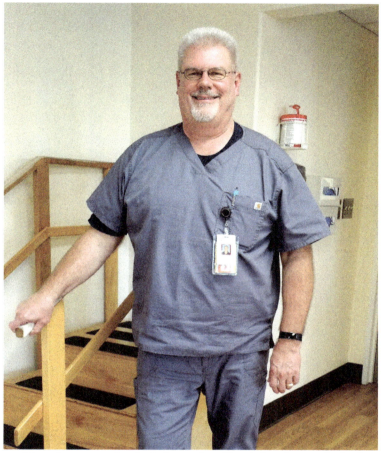

Gray Riggsbee, my physical therapist. Don't let the smile fool you.

During my time in the therapy unit, while resting in my room between sessions, I also occasionally met with Hope Duncan, the unit case manager, who also happened to be a guitarist and songwriter. Being a songwriter myself, I was interested to hear some of her original compositions, which she was willing to share. Though I was not in the condition to be an active participant, I enjoyed listening to her and thinking of the time I would once again be writing songs with others.

My time with Hope provided me a brief glimpse into regaining my normalcy.

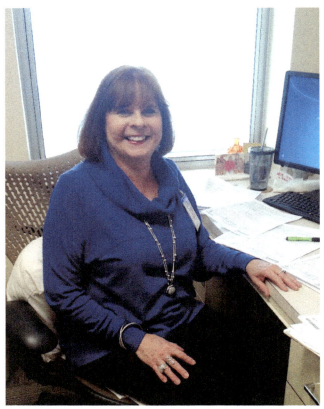

Hope Duncan, case manager and songstress.

Day 18

URING MY STAY IN THE rehab unit, I met many other stroke survivors who were at varying stages of recovery and with varying attitudes. You learn a lot when you spend time with other stroke survivors. My most startling discovery was meeting individuals who had suffered their second and third stroke and were undergoing recovery for a second or third time. I was alarmed and thought to myself, "*You mean this could happen again?*" I could not fathom that possibility and became even further motivated to overcome this stroke, and ensure that I never experienced this again.

As I said, lifestyles as well as attitudes among stroke survivors seemed to vary wildly... from the determined to the indifferent. The most bizarre example I encountered was a man who had suffered his third stroke. Yet as he spoke, he clutched a pack of cigarettes in his hands, complaining how this was supposed to be one of the leading hospitals in the country, but did not have a smoking room anywhere on the premises.

He failed to see the irony of his argument.

I was struck by how some patients were resigned and seemingly indifferent to the possibility of a second or third stroke. Their attitude seemed to be that fate was the only determinant. If a second or third stroke occurred, they appeared to believe, it was meant to be. I knew I was naïve to much that was happening around me, but I clearly believed a second or third stroke was avoidable. That is when I began to formulate my premise that it's all about the work.

Those that seemed to believe a second or third stroke was not only possible, but perhaps inevitable, obviously did not subscribe to my belief. Either I was more naïve than I thought, or they were clearly wrong. I believed then and continue now to hold to my premise that the long hard journey of recovery was and is about the work, and also the key to preventing multiple strokes.

There were others, thankfully, that did share my mindset. One patient in the unit, who became an adjunct member to the fraternity in which I had found myself, was a man named Frederick Blair. The first noticeable distinction I detected with Frederick was his ability to use both arms to navigate his wheelchair. That was a big deal to those of us who now had the use of only one arm. It was only on the occasion when he casually rolled into my room in his wheelchair to introduce himself that I learned he had not suffered a stroke, but a broken back. He had fallen from a tree, while in a deer stand, and had suffered a back and spinal injury. He had the added complication of having had back surgery to repair his discs, in addition to the rehabilitation process of relearning how to walk.

Though we had suffered different afflictions, we shared many of the same symptoms. And more importantly, we shared a similar journey and had the same attitude about how to navigate that journey.

It was my time with Frederick that reinforced the importance of attitude and determination, and that the victory was largely dependent on how hard you're willing to work. I had my second fraternity brother and lifelong friendship, born out of incidents neither of us would have chosen.

Attitude and work.

WHEN MY THERAPY SESSIONS FIRST began, I had not fully appreciated the toll the stroke had taken on my body. Though therapists are accustomed to working with patients in their weakest state, I was not accustomed to performing so poorly. I had a long way to go, and was once again reminded that the pace of recovery would be slow. I had to constantly tell myself that my job was simply to do the work, as hard and as fast as my body would allow.

From my stay in the hospital, my appreciation for the nursing staff and the therapists had grown exponentially. My appreciation for doctors, supposedly the masters of the health care domain, was not quite the same. I saw them rather infrequently, and when I did, their check-ins were brief and rather impersonal. The nurses and therapists I dealt with tended to be focused on me and my needs. Doctors, in contrast, seemed to be focused more on data related issues more than me as a human being... my chart, my blood pressure, how long before my discharge, etc. They were more like administrators rather than doctors and I certainly did not develop the same relationship with them as I did with the nurses and therapists. In fact, I had more of a relationship with the cleaning crew than I did the doctors.

This is not to say that doctors were not essential to my recovery. I assumed they were the decision-makers behind the scenes, giving directions and monitoring results. If that was true, they were certainly less visible in doing so, and far less personal. Like in many businesses, it seems the higher you are in the pecking order, the less time you spend with customers or patients. Many industries were attempting to remedy that quandary. I was unsure if the healthcare industry was doing the same. I felt the same about the health administrators and many technicians I encountered along the way. I assumed they, too, were instrumental in my recovery. They were simply less visible.

In my past life, much of my career was spent analyzing the quality of service different individuals provide. We always made it a point to preach that senior level executives should never lose touch with their customers. Doctors, I concluded, could take a page from that book.

In general, the care I received while in the hospital was excellent, with the highest marks obviously going to the nursing staff and therapists. The medical community, however much we complain about the expense or bureaucracy, got me through the most difficult period of my life, and I am eternally grateful.

CHAPTER 3
My Father

MY FATHER WAS THE PROTOTYPICAL southern male of the early 20th century. He was born in 1913 and grew up in the midst of the depression, a time when the issue of healthcare arose only if you had an emergency or were on your deathbed. Doctors were an expense few could afford and the concept of preventive medicine had yet to be established. If you took care of yourself, he believed, doctors or hospitals were unneeded. He carried those same habits and attitudes into his adult life. He was self-reliant, industrious and entrepreneurial. Though we seldom discussed politics, it was clear that his views were conservative. He relied on no one but himself for his well-being and expected everyone else to do the same.

He grew up with the misfortune of never knowing his own father. He had been abandoned by his father when he was still in the womb. My grandmother was seven months pregnant with my father when her husband left for a business trip, and never returned.

As a result, my father grew up under the tutelage of my grandmother and many aunts, uncles, and cousins. Despite those circumstances, he seemed to enjoy a pleasant and uneventful childhood and cultivated the art of drawing at an early age. He started his own sign business at the age of 19, which he called Signart Displays, and worked six and seven days a week to make it a success up until that fateful day he died of a stroke at age 70.

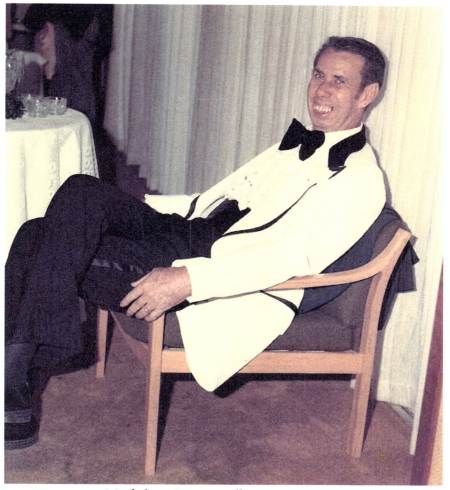

My father, George Kelly Sr. Circa 1974

Though it seems strange to say it now, he seemed to enjoy good health throughout his life. He did endure a bout with colon cancer in the 1970's. He survived at a time when survival of colon cancer was not as prevalent as it is today. Other than that, his health seemed to be the least of his issues.

He and my mother raised 10 children, and both worked full time to keep us fed, clothed and educated. As we grew older, my nine brothers and sisters and I often looked back and wondered how our parents accomplished what they did. Neither medical technology nor the means for regular health checkups were as available or as routine in the 1950's and 60's as they are today.

Like our parents, the 10 of us grew up with relatively good health and viewed healthcare either as an annual visit, a trip to the emergency room, or a matter of life and death. The concept of preventive healthcare and routine checkups had become more commonplace when we were growing up, but the habits and attitudes of our parents seemed to prevail.

Had my father been more cognizant of his health, perhaps he and we would have better known and understood his risks of a stroke, and the implications it would hold for him and his 10 children. A couple of months prior to his death from the 'big one', he had experienced a series of 'mini strokes', or TIA's as they are commonly known. Though we do not know this to be true, we believe that he only casually adhered to the warnings, and only occasionally took the medication that had been prescribed for him. All the warning signs of what was to come were there…

… as were the genes that would impact his children's lives.

I did not experience the series of mini-strokes that my father did, and had been lulled into the belief that I had no physical predictors of a stroke, and therefore never considered myself a risk. I was a distance runner and led a healthy lifestyle. I was only conceptually aware that family history was a vital indicator, if not the most vital indicator of what would be my condition. I knew very little of my father's condition and, at the time, did not appreciate the role that family history plays in our own health.

At the time of my stroke, I had no other physical indicators of what was to come. High blood pressure, high cholesterol, diabetes, overweight, smoking are all critical factors that lead to a stroke, however, I possessed none of those. The only two remaining factors were stress and family history. I assumed my stress level was as my friends and family would describe it, very low. That leaves family history.

I do not, by any means, blame my father for my stroke, but there is no question that his history affected my plight. That information is of little consolation to those of us who have already experienced a stroke, but for those who have yet to suffer this malady, heed the warning. Research your family history and your conditions, and if you find a stroke somewhere in your past, take whatever precautions are available.

End of sermon.

CHAPTER 4
Family and Friends

A S I SAID, I AM from a big family… one of 10 children. As of this writing, our family has a total of 100 brothers, sisters, wives, husbands, children, nieces, nephews, and grandchildren within our immediate family. And we all remain close. Needless to say, my family members were alarmed at the news of my stroke.

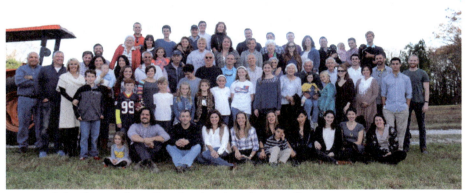

Members of my family. A critical part of my support group.

Each of them was concerned for me, and I in turn, was concerned for what it might mean for them. As previously indicated, we have some history. A brother-in-law and younger nephew had suffered strokes and seemed to recover nicely, but other than the two of them, I was the first direct descendent in our family to be impacted by our history. My fear is that I may not be the last.

As I communicated and corresponded more and more with my family and friends, I found my attitude gradually shifting about letting people know of my condition. My initial reaction after my stroke had been to downplay the event and certainly not broadcast what had happened. The more I felt the support of my family, however, the more I had become comfortable sharing what had happened. I took a phrase from the profession of architects, that says, "If you can't hide it, feature it." The love and support of my family was the catalyst for me to no longer downplay what had occurred.

I had once feared that people would perceive me differently, and was hesitant to let others know of my condition. The reactions of my friends was just the opposite. Instead of judging me or viewing me as being somehow less than perfect, they embraced me and my condition and became staunch supporters of my recovery. Perhaps I had underestimated the human condition of both my family and friends.

I was reminded that everyone experiences some form of predicament or malady at some point in their lives, and that everyone could relate in some fashion with my predicament. I found myself at times very emotional when thinking about the love and support I received from others. The more I felt it, the more motivated I was to recover, as much for myself as for everyone that was in my corner and closely monitoring my results. I wanted to succeed for them as well as myself.

I had always appreciated coming from a large family, but now it began to mean something altogether different. I was now engaged in my recovery not only for myself, but for my family. I remember years back when a brother-in-law underwent heart surgery and how the family rallied around him. I remembered how one of my sisters had recently gone through a bout with breast cancer and how everyone was focused on her recovery. I realized that we had our own dedicated support group, and how helpful that was to recovery. It was now my turn, and did I appreciate it. I now knew the power of my family's support and, boy did I need it.

Day 23

IT WAS THE DAY OF THE national football championship game between Clemson and Alabama. The Clemson quarterback, Deshaun Watson, was a native of Gainesville and a hometown hero. As a result, for many in the hospital, this was more than just a national championship game. One of the lead nurses, also named Jennifer, was particularly enthused about the game, and arranged for us to have a football party in the lobby to enjoy watching the game on television. The popcorn and the ice cream flowed. All that was missing was the beer.

As the days progressed, I had come to know the staff well, as they had me. I had been in the hospital for over three weeks. I began to realize it's never a good thing when you've been in the hospital so long that you find yourself partying with the staff. I had gotten to know them well, and appreciated all they had done for me, but it was clearly time to go home.

My family had rallied to me in a big way. I had never had a circumstance quite like this and I don't know that I have ever felt the true love and support the way I experienced from my family. First and foremost, my three children stepped up as any parent would hope their children would do. They were on the phone with one another constantly in the aftermath of my stroke and while I was still immobile at the hospital, they were shaping plans for my return home. They, and my former wife, Brenda, had already mapped out my visitation schedule and were preparing a caretaker schedule for when I came home. They all worked in close concert with my girlfriend, Jennifer, to determine who would stay with me on what days when I returned home. My support group crossed the barriers of marital status and location. They all rallied to my cause. I jokingly expressed that I had little say in the decisions being made about my life. They had taken charge, and I gladly relented.

Beyond my immediate family, my brothers and sisters were equally active. They provided a steady stream of visitors while I was in the hospital and would continue to do so when I came home. Though I was not in the best of physical condition to receive company, I welcomed seeing them and found myself motivated by their visits. I was anxious to measure my progress and their continual visits provided benchmarks for that progress.

For the first few weeks after I returned home, I enjoyed a series of homecomings with my brothers and sisters and their families.

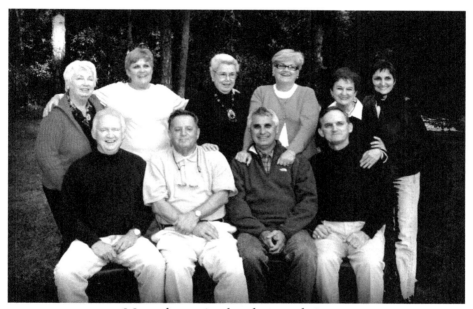

Me and my nine brothers and sisters.
Front row: Me, Bill, Pete, Mike.
Back row: Phoebe, Jackie, Kitty, Emaline, Paula and Pat.

They were welcomed sights. One of my sisters, and her husband, daughter and son-in-law, were all dog lovers, and had secretly stuffed their favorite dachshund in a handbag, to bring the added joy of a family pet into my hospital room.

Another sister and her husband brought both emotional and spiritual relief. They brought a Bible which I enjoyed reading, especially during my 2 and 3 AM moments of solitude.

As previously stated, my extended family currently numbers 100 and each of them made their presence felt throughout my recovery. Either by visitation, cards, letters, emails or text messages or some other means of communicating their love and support, never have I felt that love and support as much as I did the days following my stroke.

Although they lived as far away as Jacksonville, Florida, and Kitty Hawk. North Carolina, they were there in support of their brother. Between visits, cards, letters and emails, I felt the full love and support of my family, which was vital to my recovery.

The same can be said of friends.

Initially, I had been reluctant to spread the news of my situation, especially in the early days not knowing the true state of my condition. Many of my friends and acquaintances were completely in the dark about my circumstance. I am a proud man and found it difficult to let my friends know that I was in a weakened condition. But as the days progressed and the status of my condition was better known, I began to share more and more and the word eventually began to spread.

To some, my situation may have been little more than an item of a news update, but to my surprise and full appreciation, the true colors of my friends began to surface in the form of their love and gracious support.

Perhaps of all the friends that supported me, none did so as much as the fellow survivors I had met in the hospital, in therapy sessions, or in support groups. They were now my brothers and sisters in arms, and the only ones who truly understood what each other was experiencing. Steve Burrell suffered a stroke a week before me, and became my guide for what to expect during my recovery process. We seemed to be traveling the same path, one week apart. Frederick Blair, provided a voice of sanity during an insane time, as did many others that were traveling the same journey. Yolanda Giddens, who may have been the oldest among us, proved that age is just a number. She was a child of World War II, but showed more spunk than any of us. They, like me, had experienced the same event in some fashion. And they, like me, found themselves navigating the same rigorous road of recovery. And they were all there to cheer for the progress of their brothers and sisters in arms. Like mine, their stories bore a familiar refrain... it seemed to be all about the work. Okay, maybe work and attitude.

CHAPTER 5
AIDS, Polio, Cancer and Strokes

THERE HAVE BEEN MANY MALADIES that have plagued our society over the years that have been viewed as death sentences. From cancer, to polio, to AIDS, to strokes, the mere sound of the words would strike fear into many. Though medical technology and the human spirit have caught up, and in some cases, surpassed many of those dreaded diseases, the stigma still seemed to persist.

Prior to becoming one of the greatest presidents in our nation's history, Franklin Delano Roosevelt, at the age of 39, suddenly and inexplicably lost his ability to walk. After being examined by the leading doctors in the land using the best technology available at the time, as the world watched with grave concern, he was eventually diagnosed with a disease called polio. Suddenly, the incidence of polio was brought to the forefront of the country's consciousness, and fears and perceptions of the dreaded disease, which were already rampant, spread like wildfire throughout the country.

This was one of the many diseases and ailments that were viewed by the general public as either a death sentence or one resulting in some form of disability. In the early and mid-part of the 20th century, the word 'polio' was a dreaded sound. Known more formally as poliomyelitis, the disease struck fear in the heart of every parent. Though many people actually fully recovered, the perception existed.

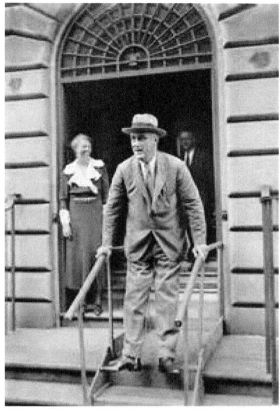

Franklin Roosevelt, wearing his braces.

Of those that experienced the disease, about 2 to 5% of children and 15 to 30% of adults perished. Another 25% experienced minor symptoms such as fever and sore throat and up to 5% reported headache, neck stiffness and pains in the arms or legs. Most people were back to normal within one or two weeks. Today the disease is fully preventable with the polio vaccine.

AIDS is a more recent example. The human immunodeficiency virus infection and acquired immune deficiency syndrome (HIV/AIDS) is a spectrum of conditions caused by infection with the human immunodeficiency virus (HIV). The disease is spread primarily by unprotected sex, contaminated blood transfusions, hypodermic needles, and from mother to child during pregnancy, delivery, or breast-feeding. In the year 2015 alone, over 36 million people were living with HIV, resulting in over 1 million deaths. Most of those lived in sub-Saharan Africa. By 2014, AIDS was estimated to have caused more than 39 million deaths. The disease has had a great impact on society, both as an illness and a source of discrimination.

When it was first discovered, it was viewed as a certain death sentence, and anyone that contracted the dreaded disease was doomed to deteriorate and ultimately die from it. That is no longer the case. Medical science and researchers have caught up with the disease, and though they have not eradicated it, they have at least arrested it.

On Nov. 7, 1991, Los Angeles Lakers point guard Earvin "Magic" Johnson shocked the world when he announced that he had contracted HIV, the virus that causes AIDS. After the press conference, the perception was that Johnson had just announced his own death sentence. Yet, 20 years later, the now-52-year-old Johnson seems to be going as strong as ever in his roles as a sports analyst, businessman and HIV activist. Who would believe in 1991, when most people believed that HIV/AIDS led to death at a young age, this outcome might have seemed possible?

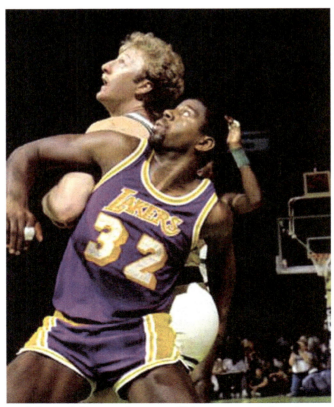

Magic Johnson, in one of his many epic battles
with Boston Celtics forward Larry Bird.

Magic Johnson has lived with the AIDS virus for more than 20 years. He is the most public example of the advances that have been made in the disease and in the treatment of it. There are thousands in this country who have the disease, yet live normal healthy lifestyles today. Though there is currently no cure or effective HIV vaccine, there is effective treatment consisting of a wide array of therapies and treatments.

Cancer, the 'Big C', has possibly been the biggest and most prevalent culprit of all. While many have experienced the dreaded disease, or had family members who have experienced it, fortunately we hear the term 'cancer survivor' more and more frequently. In fact, the American Society of Clinical Oncology recently published a list of 17 major advances in clinical cancer research, considered to be practice-changing. Further, they highlight some 70 "notable advances" that are promising towards wiping out the disease.

"Consistent, significant achievements are being made in oncology care with novel therapeutics, even in malignancies that have previously had few treatment options, as well as in defining factors that will predict response to treatment." ASCO's report goes on to distil the most significant of these advances that will positively affect the lives of cancer patients today, according to Bruce Roth, MD, co-executive editor of the report.

Cancer remains a challenge, and tragically kills more than 500,000 people in the United States every year, but the advances being made are dramatic. The 'C' word is still perhaps the scariest medical term of all, but no longer carries the same frightening stigma it once did.

To a lesser extent, strokes suffer a similar reputation. The outcome is typically viewed by many as either death or some form of debilitation. My father died of a stroke, and there is virtually no one who doesn't know of someone who has either died of a stroke or who has suffered from its occurrence today.

My biggest fear in sharing my story was that people would have that perception about me and my situation. My thought was that anyone that heard the word 'stroke' would believe that it meant I would be a changed man with a lessening of my lifestyle, or even on the brink of death. While there is no doubt my stroke did change me in many ways, I was determined that my physical ability would not be one of them. I had no intent of it negatively affecting my lifestyle. It was important to me that people viewed this as merely a temporary inconvenience. Further, I wanted people to know that the same healthy lifestyle that I and other stroke survivors knew before, was still available to us, assuming we were willing to do the work.

As I continued to test my premise that it's all about the work, I was cautioned that some stroke survivors have other factors to contend with that may not simply be remedied through hard work. I fully recognize there are many variables that impact the outcome of a stroke, such as age, the severity of the stroke, cognitive abilities that may or may not have been affected, and prior health, all of which influence the outcome of the stroke.

It can be argued for example, the attitude of a 95-year-old survivor may be different than the attitude of a 50-year-old survivor. The 95-year-old may conclude there is less life remaining and therefore willing to accept a lesser lifestyle as the natural byproduct of aging, as opposed to the 50-year-old. The opposite, which I witnessed firsthand, can also be true. While in the hospital, I met a man in his 90's who had suffered his second stroke, yet was bright and cheerful, doing his exercises willingly and enthusiastically, and another in his 50's who remained virtually comatose during his therapy, and was more interested in the smoking room then the gymnasium.

The lesson for me was age is truly just a number and the chronological age of an individual is less important than the attitude of the individual. Attitude, it appeared, was as essential as doing the work.

Prior health is another of the uncontrollable factors that can lead to a stroke. If before your stroke, you were a sedentary couch potato, the work might be more intensive than if you were a healthy physical specimen. That argument does not refute that it's all about the work. It simply suggests that some work may be harder, and take longer than others. It still comes back to doing the work.

The uncontrollable factor that may go beyond simply doing the work is the severity of the stroke or if cognitive abilities were affected by the stroke. I will not sit in judgment of anyone who has endured this malady. I simply argue that, once we have survived, the burden is ours to work as hard as we can, as long as we can and as fast as we can, to achieve a full recovery. The road may be a long and hard one, but it is ours to navigate.

CHAPTER 6
Going Home

Day 24

AFTER ALMOST A MONTH OF hospitalization and in-house therapy, I was finally discharged to go home. In that transition, I would face a four-pronged battle... My right leg and my ability to stand and walk remained limited. My right arm, hand and shoulder continued to be a challenge. My slurring speech and drooping jaw remained evident. And perhaps most importantly, I faced the challenge of fighting off the frustration and impatience that I invariably encountered.

And, to make matters worse, I was going home utterly exhausted.

More than anything, my discharge from the hospital meant I would be able to sleep in my own bed, a luxury I looked forward to with a great deal of enthusiasm. Given the constant bed checks and checks of vital signs every three hours, there was little time to actually sleep in the hospital. After nearly a month, I had my first opportunity to sleep in own bed, on my own schedule and for as long as my body would allow. And sleep I did. The first couple of days, I barely got out of bed. I thought I should be spending my time doing exercises, but the exhaustion had taken over. My body was in dire need of rest and I was only too happy to comply. I had no job to go to and my writing obligations were on hold. So, now was the perfect opportunity to let my body rest.

I came home in a wheelchair but was determined not to use it. Since it was a rental, I turned it in within the first month, determined to graduate to a less intrusive walking aid. That would be what is commonly referred to as a walker, a four-pronged device with wheels on the front and usually tennis balls on the back legs. While I found that to be helpful in navigating around the house, it gave me the sensation of being in a retirement village in South Florida. I was determined not to use it outside the house. I was desperately trying to hold on to any remaining dignity I had left.

Outside the home, my device of choice was what is referred to as a quad-cane, a walking cane with 4 feet. It was both supportive but less intrusive, and I thought did not project the same image of using a walker. By the end of February, I had graduated to a single point cane, and was even walking occasionally without the aid of any device. It was not pretty or elegant but it provided me some semblance of progress. It was important, however, as my therapists continued to remind me, progress should not be at the expense of quality or safety. I continued to have the challenge of smoothing out my stride and not walking with any form of a noticeable limp.

My arm, hand and shoulder were a different matter. While I experienced a degree of progress in the use of my hand, I had begun to feel pain in my shoulder which limited my arm movement. Almost 3 months after my stroke, I found myself still heavily reliant on my left hand to execute any type of quality movement. On selective occasions, I would use my right hand to eat and perform other tasks, but it was not pretty. Though I was right-handed I had by this time developed enough proficiency with my left hand that it almost became natural to eat and perform other tasks with my left hand. Again I was cautioned by my therapists not to abandon my right hand and become too reliant on my left. However elegant or inelegant it may have been, I had to continue to force the use of my right hand if I were to regain my normalcy.

Out of all the parts of my body, my speech was deemed the least effected by my stroke. I had a moderate degree of slurring of my speech and the right side of my mouth continued to droop. Those were features that were important to me, but given my other challenges, seemed to be a less urgent matter. That is until I saw myself. After seeing a photograph of myself in which my mouth was decidedly slanted to one side, I realized how much work I had to do to eliminate any detection of my stroke from my facial expression or speech impairments.

The team of in-house therapists had done their jobs. They were the equivalent of boot camp. The task of continuing my therapy would transition to a new, equally competent and caring team, which would now be performed on outpatient basis.

Emotionally, I was doing OK, but I still had my battles. My cognitive ability had been minimally impacted by my stroke, and that certainly helped me maintain a good attitude. But privately I experienced bouts of frustration and impatience. I had been warned on several occasions of the possibilities of depression following a stroke, so I knew I would have to fight off any negative thoughts that entered my head.

I can do this. One step at a time...

Day 40

MY RECOVERY WAS TAKING LONGER than I had hoped. I was told to expect a 3 to 6 month recovery, and though I had yet to reach three months, I was not happy with my results. I had naïvely given myself a target of 45 days to be back to normal. It seems I was the only one operating on that timeframe, and on many occasions, I appeared to be the only person not satisfied with my progress.

During my recovery, many family members and friends commented on seeing changes in my personality. My children commented that I was easier to talk to, more 'in the moment', more present. Perhaps it was my efforts to block out all distractions that might hinder my recovery. Perhaps it was my increased appreciation for life as a result of what I had gone through. Regardless of the reasons, while I was somewhat surprised, I was appreciative and happy about their conclusions.

Some of the changes, however, weren't so positive in nature. I, myself, noticed changes in my attitude and emotions regarding the world around me, and my sudden lack of motivation for anything other than that which would affect my stroke. The only reason I could write this book was because of its relationship to the stroke. I had become insular in my thoughts and suddenly uninterested in the outside world that I used to consider so important to my life.

Prior to my stroke, for example, I was a political junkie. I was in tune with all things politics. But the historical election of Donald Trump had just taken place, and yet now it seemed unimportant to me. I had lost all interest in the election that was all the news to the rest of the world. I used to be informed about all things going on around me. They now seemed to matter less.

Also before my stroke, I was passionate about NFL football, and in particular the New England Patriots. Having lived in Boston for 25 years, I was an avid sports fan and almost fanatical about the Patriots, Red Sox,

Celtics, and Bruins. Boston is a sports crazy town and that craziness certainly rubbed off on me and my children. But now I found myself only moderately enthused about the Patriots' Super Bowl win. I was certainly happy they won, but the victory and celebration seemed less meaningful than their earlier Super Bowl victories. As much as I enjoyed seeing Roger Goodell hand over the Super Bowl trophy to Robert Kraft, his adversary because of the 'deflate gate', the ceremony was not as fulfilling as it would have been otherwise. I was now focused on more important things.

I was also distracted by others around me when I walked. Especially noisy children during times when I was attempting to navigate a small area. Once a joy to me before my stroke, they were now a distraction and a nuisance that potentially impeded my progress. When I walked, I needed the entire space to myself. The presence of others, either directly in front or in my peripheral vision, represented a complication or potential distraction to my task at hand. It seemed I could only focus on one thing at a time. And that was re-learning how to live.

Along with my physical abilities, I seemed to have lost much of my tolerance and patience. I attributed these changes to my singular focus in carrying out the basic task before me, such as walking, or my focus on my recovery. I was now indifferent to the outside world and now only focused on one thing… my recovery. The things that mattered so much to me before my stroke now mattered very little. I had a job to do.

I was uncontrollably emotional at the time. I would cry at the drop of a hat, especially if the topic related to my family in some way. Steve Burrell, one of my fellow stroke survivors, shared the same sensation. He once commented jokingly, "If someone said 'watermelon' or 'butterfly' I would cry." I could relate. My emotions, like his, were laid bare for all to see.

I learned that it was common for strokes to affect your emotions, and your filter. Before my stroke, I was somewhat careful and usually politically correct about what I said in public. I now found myself blurting out on any particular subject. If I saw it or thought it, I said it, and many times with little or no concern about the subject or what or who it may pertain to.

Humor was no different. I found myself laughing out loud uncontrollably over the least little thing, many times at myself and the absurdity of my situation. Many times I was amused by the snail-like pace of my walk with a walker or cane. My common refrain was, "I'm coming, I'm coming." I felt like the old man character played by Tim Conway on the Carol Burnett Show. My outbursts were uncontrollable and unpredictable, and in many cases, humorous. It was if I had some form of Tourette's syndrome.

Laughter, tears, and uncontrollable outbursts appeared to be hallmarks of my new personality.

My transition from the hospital to home also meant I had to develop a whole new routine. While in the hospital, it was very structured. Meals, medication, therapy, and rest time all had a sense of regimentation. When I came home, however, I had to develop my own routine. I no longer had nurses and therapists to take care of my every need. And my needs were many. The burden of caregiving had now shifted to family members and friends. The simplest matters of opening a jar, or going from the bed to the coffee table and sofa, or getting dressed, were matters that required some degree of assistance, and, thankfully, I had family members or friends there to assist me.

I did not enjoy being dependent on others, even when they were more than happy to help. I know of no stroke patient, or for that matter, anyone that enjoys being waited on. All we want to do, I thought, was to be fully functioning human beings without having to rely on others. The goal of being independent was a major motivating factor for me. I was determined to become fully independent as quickly as possible. I no longer had alarms on my bed or wheelchair, as I did in the hospital, so I was now able to move around more freely. The simple question was how quickly could I improve to do certain tasks for myself and no longer rely on others to do them for me?

Though I disliked the notion, I was eternally grateful for the round-the-clock care provided by Jennifer, my three children, my former wife, Brenda, and other family members and friends. They saw me in my worst moments and seemed to accept them without complaint. I know that much of what I endured can be equated to aging, which inevitably confronts each of us. But I was not yet ready to succumb to that inevitability. I was not yet ready to inflict my inability to function on another human being. I was independent before my stroke and was determined to gain that same level of independence after my stroke.

Once home, I also had a flurry of doctor's appointments and medical follow-ups to take care of. Among others, I saw my primary care physician, Dr. Chenard, who had only recently learned of my stroke upon my discharge. He, like me, was dumbfounded by what had happened. In all my previous checkups over the past two years, my vital signs had been in the normal range … no apparent warning signs. Since my vital signs were all deemed to have been good, we both surmised that my family history or stress were the most likely culprits. And he, like me, was eager to find out. He was as curious and eager as me, to find out what had happened and do what was necessary to facilitate my recovery.

My therapies remained the centerpiece of my recovery and were now being continued on an outpatient basis three and four days a week. They consisted of exercises that continued to test my capabilities. As my movement improved, so did the exercises become more intense. They were grueling. My endurance was slowly beginning to also improve, so the exhaustion was beginning to lessen, but the sessions were intense nonetheless. They were an extension of what I was doing in the hospital, only on a more intensive basis and with the use of more toys and under the guidance of a new team of therapists.

My physical therapy was now being led by a young, California-transplanted therapist named Peter Park and a formidable group of women named Denise Filush, Valerie Gohman, and Katie Wallace. My occupational therapy was led by a spry, British woman named Joanna Osbahr. The challenge of helping me eliminate the sagging of my mouth and speaking more clearly now belonged to Rebecca Sabo and Donna Brooks. This team of professionals had become my new lifeline and continued what the in-house therapists had begun. If my hospital therapy was my boot camp, I was now in advanced training.

Compared to my initial days in the hospital when I was barely able to stand, I was dramatically improved, but still had a long way to go. While my ability to walk had progressed, the new exercises demonstrated how limited it was. As in the hospital, I was continually humbled by new and more challenging exercises. A slight moment of cockiness achieved by some small victory, invariably turned to a rapid dose of humility with the introduction of a new, more demanding exercise.

Victory was not yet in sight.

Peter, Denise, Valerie and Katie continued the physical therapy that Gray had begun in the hospital. The exercises now were less about being able to stand or walk across the room, which was my challenge in the hospital, and more about improving the pace and stride of my walk. I had completely forgotten what my normal walk looked or felt like, so my therapy sessions were an exercise in relearning what would before be taken for granted. I had to mentally think through and completely relearn my leg movements, my arm movements, and the normal rotation of my shoulders as I walked.

How much shoulder turn do you engage in as you walk? To those who enjoy the ability to walk naturally, that is something you never have to think about. You just do it. But when your brain has to be rewired, it is as much a mental exercise as it is physical.

My occupational therapy, begun in the hospital by Niki and Charlie, was now the responsibility of Joanna. While in the hospital, I was limited in my ability to move my right arm and shoulder, but at least there was no pain associated with the effort. The shoulder was still numb from the paralysis, so whatever pain existed had not yet begun to register. By the time I began meeting with Joanna, I was feeling the pain. It had begun to register in my brain. I was now dealing with the dual challenge of a lack of mobility and pain. It felt as if I had digressed, but over a period of weeks, I had begun to experience some progress with the use of my arm.

I also continued to work on my speech, which I had begun in the hospital with Jen. That task now fell to Rebecca, with help from Donna. Though deemed to be the least of my challenges, there was still work to be done in that area. I still occasionally slurred my words and my mouth remained slanted to one side. Our goal was to work on refining both my ability to articulate clearly and eliminate the droop in my lip. As Jen had told me on many occasions before, this would be a long process. Rebecca and Donna reinforced that message, and the results gradually began to show.

My therapy was my job. I went to therapy as one would go to work every day, but the work did not in there. In each therapy session, I learned new exercises or a new muscles to concentrate on in my recovery efforts, but to realize the desired results, I would have to repeat those exercises endlessly when at home. Like going to school, homework was a necessity and as critical as the therapy sessions themselves. It seemed my hardest work was occurring between therapy sessions.

As with the group of therapists in the hospital, I forged a tight bond with my outpatient therapists. In addition to my physical recovery, they were instrumental in helping me maintain my emotional equilibrium at a time when my progress was seemingly happening at a snail's pace in my frustration was evident. They were dedicated to finishing what the hospital therapists had begun, and had their hands full in doing so. And like all the other healthcare professionals I encountered, they excelled at their jobs and showed the same level of professionalism and personal care as those in the hospital.

The journey continued.

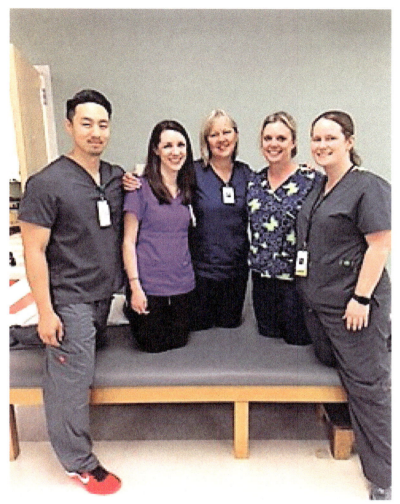

My Outpatient Therapy Team:
L to R: Peter Park, Rebecca Sabo, Joanna Osbahr,
Valerie Gohman, Denise Filush.
Not Pictured: Donna Brooks and Katie Wallace.

The periodic assessments conducted during my therapy sessions continued to show moderate improvement, though certainly not as fast as I had hoped. It was evident I only part way back to normal. When I was not in therapy, I was at home doing exercises. My mantra remained, 'it is all about the work', and the sooner I did my exercises, I was convinced, the sooner I would return to normal. Though I had trained for marathons, and had been accustomed to 70 and 80 hour work weeks during my career, this was without question, the hardest I had ever worked in my lifetime. Largely because, this time, I was without the benefit of one side of my body. Routine movements such as raising my hand above my head was like trying to lift a 500 pound weight. My body had never been weaker, but my resolve had never been stronger.

Through it all, I was constantly reminded to rest... allow the brain time to rewire itself... allow the body time to re-learn how it is supposed to function and heal. The idea was not new to me, but it was hard to do. I was impatient and eager to keep working towards my ultimate objective. I was continually chastised by the therapy staff and my family members to rest. The idea of resting between sessions was logical, but I had difficulty factoring rest periods into my regimen. In the past, anytime I faced challenges or was backed into a corner, under any situation, my tendency was to fight... outwork the opponent. But in this case, I had to learn to give in to what had happened to me and share the workload with my body. I had to do the work, but allow the body to also do its work. I had to learn to give myself to a journey that was not of my own choosing.

If you have a cold, you can take medicine, but you also have to rest and allow the body the opportunity to recover. This was no different.

I had begun to understand the process, but it was a difficult, and seemingly counter-intuitive process to digest... Do the work, but allow yourself to give in to what has happened to you. Work, but don't fight it.

It all seemed so confusing.

Day 64

I WAS NOW ABLE TO WALK without the assistance of a cane and navigate my way around my house, though still with somewhat of a limp, and still with some degree of awkwardness. In addition, each morning, I required anywhere from 30 minutes to an hour to stretch and allow my body to warm up. My muscles and nerves were still rediscovering how to work and required time in the morning to get started. I experienced severe tightness overnight that had to loosen itself. Sometimes my early morning exercises gave me the sensation that I was back in the hospital during my earliest days of recovery. My days of optimism continued to be matched by days of frustration. It was clear that I had progressed, but it was equally clear that I was nowhere near my desired destination. I was now dependent on caregivers only for transportation, but now the caregivers were family and friends, not paid professionals.

In the spirit of full disclosure, until my stroke, the idea of caregiving and caregivers were notions I had not given much thought to. Caregiving is a broad and all-encompassing term, and covers the gamut of anything and everything required to help someone get through their day. I began to grow increasingly sensitive to how the burden of caregiving had shifted, virtually overnight, from hospital staff, who were trained and paid to perform those tasks, to the family and friends who were now giving of their time simply out of love. And they were unpaid, less experienced, and had lives of their own to contend with. It seemed so unfair. My need for caregivers had diminished, but as I witnessed the nonstop work they performed day in and day out, I remember thinking, their lives were affected by this event as much as my own. My caregivers were the lifeblood of my recovery, and I was determined to make their work as easy as possible.

I had thought about and watched the physical limitations other stroke survivors had experienced, and their need for caregivers. I realized the degree of care required varies from individual to individual, and was further aware that some survivors had professional caregivers come into the home to provide the necessary assistance. But the fact that I was most struck by, was that the jobs of caregiving, unless paid professionals, are suddenly thrust upon individuals, and many times, involuntarily. I then began to realize how that is not just true for the caregivers of stroke survivors, but the caregivers of any and all survivors, regardless of the circumstance.

I grew increasingly aware of and concerned about the notion of 'caregiver burnout', described as 'a point in which the caregiver experiences a state of physical, emotional, and mental exhaustion typically accompanied by a change in attitude... from positive and caring to negative and unconcerned.'

All of my caregivers were wonderful and I was extremely thankful, and I wanted nothing to do with being guilty of causing caregiver burnout. I began to look for ways to ensure that those who cared for me during my time of dependence, had ample opportunity to take a break from my neediness and not have them suffer from any form of caregiver burnout on my watch.

As a writer, my schedule was pretty much my own, but I did have pending projects waiting for me. I was anxious to get back to work, and eventually found my way back to my desk, but the most elementary tasks remained painful and clumsily performed. Typing was out of the question and operating a mouse with my right hand was next to impossible. I could barely reach the on/off switch of my computer, due to the limited movement in my shoulder, and had to virtually retrain myself on the operations of my PC due to my extended absence. Though I was slow and awkward, I was once again able to work. Thank goodness for talk–to–text software, which allowed me to type using my voice instead of my fingers. I would have been completely out of luck without it.

Among other projects I was working on prior to my stroke, was a workshop group that was originally scheduled to begin in January. The group had patiently agreed to reschedule the workshop to a time when my recovery would allow. We postponed the workshop for one month, knowing I would not be fully recovered, but would at least be able to adequately conduct the workshop. Again, the dictation software was invaluable as my right hand was still not functional.

I couldn't help but wonder about those who faced challenges far greater than my own.

Day 70

NOW INTO MY THIRD MONTH as a stroke survivor, I continued to ask the same question of every healthcare official I encountered, 'When will this be over? When should I expect to return to normal?' The answer predictably also remained the same … *"It all depends. Every case is different."* I had grown weary of the same maddening response. While I knew it to be true, it was maddening nonetheless. I was eager to experience a full recovery, sooner rather than later, and that just wasn't happening.

I was desperate to come up with a solution, even if it was my own. I tried everything, even some inventions of my own. I created a form of 'constraint therapy' for my lip and drooping mouth by taping the unaffected side of my face in hopes of more quickly activating the other side. I purchased a rowing machine which I incorporated into my morning exercise routine in hopes that it would expedite the recovery of my leg and arm. I purchased an inflatable sleeve to keep my arm straight during its exercises. I rigged up my quad cane to use as an arm brace to elevate my recovering arm and hand. I stood in the shower for hours on end, in hopes that the hot water would loosen up the muscles in my shoulder and legs, and even my face. I was determined to find a solution by taking the exercises from my therapy sessions, and in addition to doing those at home, I constructed my own. In the spirit of safety and full disclosure, I did advise my therapists of the various exercises I had concocted to ensure I was not inadvertently creating some unintended consequence. They assured me none of the measures I had created were causing any undue harm. They just smiled (laughed) politely, complimented my efforts, and encouraged me to keep trying. In the end, none of my special maneuvers resulted in the magical effect I was seeking, but I continued my efforts to innovate.

My family and friends continued to tell me how well I was doing, but I was still not satisfied. My recovery was not fast enough for me. I knew that my stroke was not as severe as others had experienced, and I knew I was in good health when my stroke occurred, therefore enhancing my recovery. But I had also seen people go home from the hospital in five days or less and seemingly experience a full recovery in matter of weeks, not months as mine appeared to be.

While that was not completely true, I had to continue to battle my frustration and impatience. Rationally, I knew that the recovery from a stroke is not much different than recovering from any other illness. It depends on the severity of the illness and the state of the individual, and it takes time. However rational that truth may be, I was not entirely rational during my recovery. I wanted it and I wanted it now. And nothing seemed to be happening at the pace I had anticipated or desired. There was no big 'aha' moment. There were only a series of small, moderate improvements that I could barely detect. The improvements occurred without a doubt, but they were in small and seemingly miniscule doses, and happening at a snail's pace.

That is, when there *were* improvements. More than once there were stretches of time when there seemed to be no progress at all or even some digression to a degree. There were days I found myself walking at the same level as when I had just left the hospital.

Was I going backwards? Was I digressing?

Ultimately, the answer was no. It was simply the non-linear road the human body tends to travel during its recovery. No one had bothered to explain this to me until now. While I was in hope of a straight line, my recovery seemed to be like the flight of a housefly or a bumblebee... all over the place. Three steps forward and two steps sideways, became my common response when people would ask how I was doing. Their response, in turn, was typically 'Well at least you are advancing and not going backwards.' That answer was of little consolation to me at the time.

During that time I was managing to walk unassisted... but it was still not at my normal pace or very elegant. It was also not consistent and was frowned upon by my therapists because of the risk of falling. But that seemed to be the only thing I could point to that indicated progress.

My recovery remained an exercise in mental concentration as much as physical, and again had to devise tricks to maintain my concentration. Many times, I counted aloud as I walked, and when I was not counting out loud, I was resorting to other means of focusing on my steps and my stride, such as humming. To maintain my steps and the rhythm of my pace, I would hum imaginary drum cadences, either out loud or in my head, as if I were marching. It was not uncommon for others in the room to hear me humming cadences or military counts or sounding like the drummer in a marching band as I walked.

Hup, two, three, four! Sound-off-three-four!

I HAD GROWN ACCUSTOMED TO my progress continuing at a snail's pace, and I tended to discount any signs of accomplishment for fear I would revert back to my previous level. I was not going to be satisfied until I was completely back to normal. I wanted my stride to be more elegant and consistent. I wanted to regain the full movement of my arm and shoulder. I remained dissatisfied and frustrated that I had not achieved more, and at a faster pace. In retrospect, I realize now that I failed to celebrate the small victories that would become memorable milestones in my recovery. Others saw and celebrated the progress. I would not.

I had advanced sufficiently that I could now shower and get dressed on my own, though it seemed to take forever, and it was thoroughly exhausting. There were times when I spent more than five minutes just tying my shoes. My attire remained sparse with easy-to-put-on and take-off clothes, but that, too, took much time and effort. There were times when I would sit on the bed to rest for five or 10 minutes in utter exhaustion after putting on my clothes and before embarking onto the next chore.

I was no longer the hare. I had become the tortoise!

In addition to regaining my natural motion, my major challenges continued to be my speed and my endurance, a shortcoming which were, many times, pointed out by the therapists' formal assessments. One of the exercises in physical therapy, for example, was to sit in a chair, stand up and walk 10 feet to a small cone, go around it and return to the chair. How long would that take you? My first attempt was timed at one minute. ONE MINUTE, to walk 10 feet and go around a cone, and return to sit down in the chair. And that was with the aid of a cane. The expected goal would be to reduce that time to less than 13 seconds, walking unassisted. They may as well have said, 'Then you have to do a double cartwheel across the floor and land on your feet.'

Going from one minute with a cane, to less than 13 seconds without the cane, epitomized my challenges.

Speed and endurance.

I HAD IMPROVED MY GRIP strength in my affected hand but it was still tested at less than half of what it should be. I was able to raise my arm over my head, though I did experience a moderate degree of pain in my shoulder as a result. My goal for my arm and hands was to regain the routine movements I enjoyed before my stroke. I knew that would be difficult, but that was my goal. I could no longer sign my name. I could no longer write or type. I spent endless days writing my ABCs and signing my name on a legal pad for practice. Both were completely illegible for the first few days and both were exhausting. I was left breathing as though I had just run a mile just to write my name.

I was no longer able to type with my right hand and as an author, though I had dictation software, that was a serious issue. Typing with only one hand, especially my left hand, was a slow and tedious task. I continued to attempt to re-engage my right hand on the keyboard, but I invariably had to revert to my left hand. I quickly learned that if you are accustomed to typing with two hands, which I was, your left hand does not even remember where the keys are located that you normally type with your right hand. And even with the use of dictation software, I could sit at my desk to use my computer for no more than an hour due to the exhaustion.

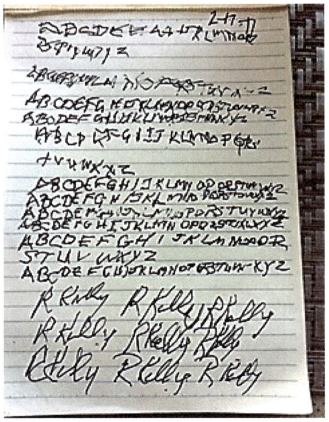

My early attempts to regain my writing ability.

Opening the refrigerator or removing lids from jars using my right hand was seemingly impossible. Anything that required both my left and right hand together was out of the question at that stage. I remember being very proud and happy the morning I picked up a cup of coffee with my right hand without spilling it.

In the privacy of family or close friends who were less critical and more forgiving of my condition, I continued to attempt to eat with my right hand. It continued to be inelegant and inconsistent, and many times very messy. When the fatigue overtook my effort, I reverted to my left-hand which by then, had become quite proficient unfortunately. Though I had developed some degree of ambidexterity, that newfound skill unfortunately revealed how little I was able to use my right hand.

In contrast to my constant frustration with my slow progress, I did manage to occasionally celebrate small victories. In my earliest days in the hospital, there were times when I would beam like a proud baby boy with the slightest of movements. I wanted to show off to my family and friends the way an infant does when they learn a new task.

"Look at me everybody. I can move my thumb!"

OH, TO PERFORM THE SIMPLE tasks I once took for granted. I so longed for them, but now knew I would have to work to regain them.

That was the nature of coming home. It was all about the work. I had a job to do. Nothing else seemed to matter.

CHAPTER 7
The Long and Winding Road

Day 76

NOTHING SEEMS TO HAPPEN AS fast or go as smoothly as you want. And it is often a lonely vigil. That is true of life and certainly true of recovering from a stroke. Instead of a linear path trending upwards, my recovery continued to resemble the flight of a bumblebee... up, down, forwards and backwards.

It was the Ides of March. I felt as if I had hit a wall. I had not regressed, but I certainly felt I was not progressing as I had hoped or expected. This was turning into a saga. Despite the grueling leg exercises I performed on a daily basis, I continued to walk with a limp and an occasional foot drag. I continued to experience pain in my shoulder and my motion continued to be limited. In the mornings and in the evenings, when I was tired or just waking up, I continued to slur my speech. My ability to write was no better. I felt like I was stuck in a rut and experienced perhaps my lowest point emotionally. While the rest of the world was focused on Donald Trump's Russian connections, my focus was more narrowly defined... on my recovery.

I had established a timeline in my head but my body was not complying. I was told by healthcare professionals that to expect, at a minimum, a 3 to 6 month recovery. I was approaching three months since my stroke and had hoped to beat those odds. I was failing. I wasn't the super achiever I had hoped to be. Perhaps I was average, after all. The Ides of March would not be the milestone I had hoped. I was disappointed and frustrated, and struggling not to allow those emotions to enter my thoughts. Back to the architect's expression, 'If you can't hide it, feature it,' I decided rather than resist the frustration, I would accept it as part of the process. *(Give yourself in to it. Don't fight it. Don't resist...)* I had to give myself to what had happened to me. I had to occasionally allow myself to have a bad day.

Oh well, so much for recovering by March. Maybe April would be my magic month.

Some two years prior to my stroke, my sister had been diagnosed with breast cancer and seemed to experience many of the same seesaw emotions. Loneliness, frustration, even brushes of depression, three steps forward and one step sideways. But she ultimately embraced her challenge and won her battle. Did cancer patients go through the same up-and-down cycle as stroke survivors?

I was beginning to rethink the fraternity I had joined. Perhaps it should not be restricted only to stroke survivors, but to any and all who had survived any malady that required such a battle. Whether strokes, breast cancer, a broken back, or some other disruption to their life, there were many who had fought or were fighting the same battle, and in many cases, battles tougher than my own.

While my progress was evident and encouraging to others around me, for me it continued to be agonizingly slow, and in small indiscernible increments. My days at home following my return from the hospital became a long road of frustration and impatience, interspersed with occasional small victories. Where were the big 'aha' moments when I would suddenly or magically begin walking smoothly? When would I have the full use of my right arm? When would the droop in my jaw suddenly disappear, and I be able to speak without slurring my words? Where was the 'voila'? That moment continued to escape me. I only had small, modest victories to celebrate. I had to work at restraining my frustration.

To make matters worse, throughout this time I occasionally experienced what I call 'The Big Tease'. Those were moments, typically when I was exercising in bed, or when I experienced some degree of normalcy in my movement. Tangible progress... a degree of normalcy... I thought I was actually nearing full recovery, when in reality, it was just a fleeting moment of relief. The next morning when I would awaken, the same stiffness and pain was there awaiting me. It was an up and down roller coaster ride, and I had to work to keep my sanity. Once again I had to curtail my frustration and accept the up's and the down's as the natural progression of recovery.

During my stay in the hospital, I was constantly reminded of the possibility of depression and how many stroke survivors experience some form of depression. Though frustrated and impatient on many occasions, I was determined not to let that happen to me. On those occasions, when I would find myself frustrated due to my lack of progress, I had to resist any negative thoughts. I had to maintain a positive focus. That was my upbringing, my DNA, and I knew how important that was to my recovery. And the last thing I needed was an appointment with a psychiatrist to go with all of my many other doctors' appointments.

I had to draw on a critical ingredient that had always kept me focused and driving forward... having a goal to work towards. I needed to have something to look forward to, something that required focus to keep me from obsessing over my stroke. Perhaps that would be the key to my recovery. I had ghostwriting projects, workshop projects and speaking engagements in addition to planned family outings awaiting my return. I had a pending 5K road race with my grandchildren, and going scuba diving with my children. I had plenty to look forward to and was determined to be able to do each of them. I had to give all the exercises I was doing a sense of purpose.

My progress continued to feel like it was going forwards, backwards, and sideways. I had to constantly remind myself that I had never actually regressed during my recovery, but there were several days when I seemed to experience no progress at all. This was taking longer than I had anticipated. I had plans. Things to do. Places to go. I didn't have time for this.

It seemed as if I were in the movie, "Groundhog Day." I seemed to keep repeating the same day over and over again. There were times when I felt no progress at all, and other times, when I felt like I was repeating the same progress I had already experienced. I assumed that was not the case, and it was reaffirmed by doctors and therapists that I was simply experiencing a lull or a plateau. I was told it was probably my body's way of telling me it needed a rest. Those were very frustrating days. I had hoped to experience a straight line of progress from week to week, and that was not the case. Three days forward and two days sideways, seemed to turn into three weeks forward and two weeks sideways.

The body heals at its own pace, and unfortunately, I was living that reality. Be patient, I was told. Give yourself to it. Take what the body gives you. Easy to say, difficult to do.

A major part of my job was keeping my attitude positive and my frustration at bay, which I did, but it remained simmering just below the surface. That is where faith kicked in. I had to believe God had his hands on me throughout my recovery. I had to believe He was guiding me through this. Many of those 3 AM conversations, when they were not with the nurses or nurse technicians, were with God.

Work, patience, attitude and faith.

MY WALKING HAD GRADUALLY IMPROVED. I had graduated from a walker, to a four-pronged cane, to a single cane and eventually, to walking completely unassisted. My stride was not yet full nor was my gate particularly attractive, but I was walking nonetheless, and at a slightly improved pace.

My shoulder and arm remained another matter. For an extended period of time, I experienced pain and stiffness in my right shoulder and was still only able to execute a few of the functions that would constitute a full arm motion. I had developed a grip in my right hand, but I learned through my therapy sessions the strength of my right hand grip was about half the strength of my left hand grip. Not good.

I was accustomed to lifting weights and when I came home from the hospital, I immediately began to incorporate weights into my daily exercise routine. I later learned that was an ill-advised move for my shoulder. Range of motion first, strength second, I was told. I was under the mistaken belief that strength was first and foremost and that was my objective. As anyone educated in shoulder issues will tell you, just the opposite is the key to regaining the use of your arm and hands.

While living in Asia, I studied the principles of war and fighting, and in particular, the art of boxing in contrast to the martial arts, such as judo or karate. What was particularly interesting was how the two concepts seemed to apply to the philosophies of life, and to my situation. Boxing is the art of overpowering your opponent with brute force. Martial arts, in contrast, is more about inviting your opponent's force into your body and using it as a lever to redirect it away from you and to your advantage. I had to remind myself to treat my challenge more like martial arts, and less like boxing. I was not going to overpower this opponent, so I had to learn to accept the force of my opponent, invite it in, and attempt to redirect it to my advantage. Learning to accept and embrace what had happened to me was a difficult but powerful lesson.

Also during my time in Asia, I had become a student of the Zen philosophy and the whole notion of 'be at one with the struggles life poses.' I have actually felt like I was more of a 'martial arts' kind of guy than a 'boxing' kind of a guy. But when my stroke occurred, it seems like my fighting instincts kicked in and I went into full attack mode. Perhaps I should have allowed my martial arts mindset to have a little more influence in the way I approached my situation.

I even wrote a song that reflected that philosophy, which I had to remind myself. I entitled it "Where the River Flows". I won't bore you with the entire song, but a portion of it tells the message:

When I was a boy I asked my dad,
Why does life seem so hard.
Sometimes it's good, and sometimes it's bad,
and sometimes it tears me apart.

He lingered for a while, then looked at me and smiled,
and this is what I heard him say:

Life seems hard son, I suppose,
But it ain't hard if you just let it go.
Trust in God son, He always knows.
Let life take you where the river flows.

Trust in God son, He always knows. Let life take you where the river flows. Perhaps I knew something when I wrote those lyrics. Work hard, and let the chips fall where they may. Let the river flow. In my eagerness to improve, I had temporarily forgotten my own message.

I replaced my strength training in my arms with stretching exercises. Though, I must admit that through it all, I continued to ponder when would I be able to resume my daily strength exercise regimen including my hand weights and my heavy ropes? The weakness in my shoulder and arms was evident, and I was eager to correct it. But stretching had become a crucial component at this stage of my recovery. My limitations were a result of tightness as much as weakness.

Sometimes I would use my remaining good hand (my left) to guide my right in a series of stretching exercises. To my surprise and amazement, there were times when much of the soreness I was experiencing in my shoulder was temporarily remedied by stretching. Had I discovered something new? Had I come up with a new technique which needed to be shared with the therapeutic community? No, not really. It was simply another case of The Big Tease. My body, as well as my memory and span of concentration were simply inconsistent. Weeks before, my therapist had reminded me of the importance of stretching before strength. I simply didn't remember. My span of concentration was such that each time I rediscovered the power of stretching, I had to be reminded it is not something I had not been told or discovered before.

As I progressed, ever so slightly, I was continuing to rely on caregivers less and less for my day-to-day existence. Shortly after coming home from the hospital, I had gained my independence for bathroom related activities, but I was still delayed in performing other routine functions such as cleaning or laundry or cooking. For the first time in my life I actually looked forward to performing those menial tasks, not because I enjoyed them, but because they would serve as an indicator of my progress. I constantly sought out any indication of my progress.

Stretching and exercising remained the centerpiece of my recovery. If there was a lull in my activities, I found a way to fill it by stretching or exercising. Sometimes it was a mere matter of standing up and sitting down repeatedly. Sometimes it was walking from side to side or back and forth. Sometimes it was reaching for the sky on a repeated basis, even if it was with the assistance of my good hand. Sometimes it was folding my arms behind my head and stretching out the pain. However menial to the general population, those movements were critical to us stroke survivors, and difficult to perform.

Movement, not just stretching and exercising, I was reminded, was another key. That was a difficult lesson for me to learn about my arm and shoulder. I had been conditioned to believe that when you cannot perform a function, it is a matter of stretching and getting stronger. Instead, I had to tell my brain that my muscles were still there and yearning to relearn how to operate. While there continued to be many nights when I was up at 3 AM performing stretches or exercises, in retrospect, I may have been better off simply moving my affected body parts. I perhaps took the issue of exercise too seriously.

I was also reminded of the criticality of rest. *(Just let your body be with it; Let the river flow.)* Those periods of rest, I was reminded, are when your body recovers. I had to be reminded that finding the right balance between exercise, stretching, movement, and rest was my formula to a full recovery.

It remained all about the work… and the exercise… and the stretching… and the movement… and resting in between. This was all very confusing.

I was a slow learner.

CHAPTER 8
Unfortunately, I'm Not Alone

Another of my discoveries as a stroke survivor was how frequently strokes occur and how many people were affected by them. I didn't realize just how big a fraternity I had joined. In addition to those I had met personally, according to the National Stroke Association, someone suffers a stroke every 40 seconds and it can happen to anyone at any time. Some 200,000 cases are diagnosed each year in the United States alone, and there are projections for even higher numbers to come in the year 2017.

There were a few other stroke facts that I discovered:

- Stroke is the fifth leading cause of death in the United States, killing more than 130,000 Americans each year—that's 1 of every 20 deaths.
- A stroke, sometimes called a brain attack, occurs when a clot blocks the blood supply to the brain or when a blood vessel in the brain bursts.
- Someone in the United States has a stroke every 40 seconds. Every four minutes, someone dies of stroke.
- Every year, about 795,000 people in the United States have a stroke. About 610,000 of these are first or new strokes; 185,000 are recurrent strokes.
- Stroke is a leading cause of disability. Stroke reduces mobility in more than half of stroke survivors age 65 and over.
- Strokes costs the nation $33 billion annually, including the cost of health care services, medications, and lost productivity.
- You can't control some stroke risk factors, like heredity, age, gender, and ethnicity. Some medical conditions—including high blood pressure, high cholesterol, heart disease, diabetes, overweight or obesity, and previous stroke or transient ischemic attack (TIA)—can also raise your stroke risk.
- Avoiding smoking and drinking too much alcohol, eating a balanced diet, and getting exercise are all choices you can make to reduce your risk.

Some common warning signs and symptoms of a potential stroke are…

- Sudden numbness or weakness of the face, arm, or leg—especially on one side of the body.
- Sudden confusion, trouble speaking or understanding.
- Sudden trouble seeing in one or both eyes.
- Sudden trouble walking, dizziness, loss of balance or coordination.
- Sudden severe headache with no known cause.

Some of this I knew. Some of it was an eye-opener. The more I learned, the less enchanted I was with the new fraternity to which I now belonged. Looking for the positive in all of this, in my analysis, I came up with a proverbial good news/bad news scenario.

There are far too many strokes that take place in our society (bad news)… yet we have a growing database from which to learn about the issue, and determine how we can make it a thing of the past (good news).

In my sphere alone, there were many others who had experienced the same or a similar predicament, which they were willing to share. Some of them, I have already referenced. Some of them are new. Here are a sampling of their stories, in their own words.

The Steve Burrell Story

(As told by Steve Burrell)

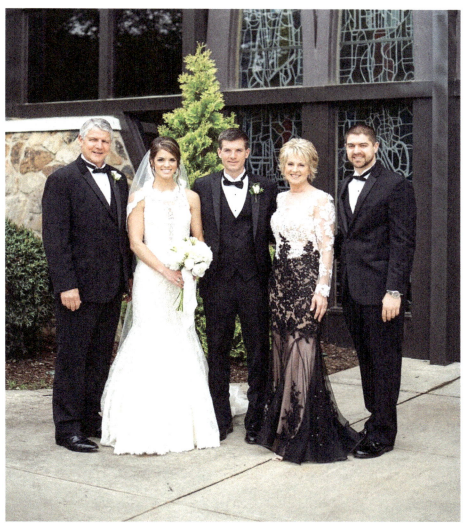

L to R: Steve, Bradee Burrell Aderholt,
Drew Aderholt, Carol Burrell, and Lee Burrell

I T WAS THURSDAY, DECEMBER 8, 2016, and I was looking forward to the weekend. I had big plans. The following Saturday, I was to referee the AAA state football championship game at the Georgia Dome in Atlanta. It would've been my second consecutive year as the "white-hat" official in the championship game. To me, it was a very big deal!

Sunday morning, Lakewood Baptist Church's Crosspoint Choir was presenting its Christmas concert, and Sheila Rogers, Kat Wofford, and I were to sing one of the specials, "Listen to the Angels Singing," by Bill and Gloria Gaither. Who wouldn't want to sing an uplifting Gaither song at Christmastime?

Sunday night, my wife Carol and I were taking Bill and Patti Risinger to Atlanta to hear the Atlanta Master Chorale at Emory University as guests of Tommy and Tammy Herrington. Bill is worship leader at Lakewood in Gainesville, Georgia.

Over just a few hours on the morning of December 8, all of those plans; the game, the concert, the Chorale—simply melted away.

I had gotten up earlier than usual that day. It was about six o'clock. I went to my office at home to watch videos of the two AAA football teams, preparing for game on Saturday. But something wasn't right about me. When I walked, I sensed a disconnection, like somebody else was walking in my body. I tried to explain the feeling to Carol, but it was hard to put into words.

Carol fixed breakfast—eggs and toast—but I couldn't eat it all. That was unusual. I told Carol I wanted to lie down for a few minutes; I had a business appointment at noon in Cumming, Georgia, and I wanted this weird feeling of disconnection to go away before I drove twenty-three miles in my truck. After about thirty minutes, I got up, took a shower and got dressed. I actually seemed a little better, but I still felt weird.

Driving to Cumming, I noticed I couldn't grip the steering wheel very well with either hand and I ran off the road a couple of times. Then I became nauseated. I stopped the truck and telephoned my boss to tell him I wasn't feeling well, and wouldn't make the luncheon. I noticed my speech was slurred; it was like my tongue was really thick.

I drove back home, about seven miles away, still feeling like I had no grip in my hands. I walked into the house. I didn't walk fast, but at least I was walking. I sat down in a chair and called our daughter, Bradee, a registered nurse in the Intensive Care Unit at the Northeast Georgia Medical Center near downtown Gainesville. She was busy, so my call went to voice mail. I called Carol, who is President and CEO of the medical center. That call also went to voice mail.

Bradee discovered this message, sent at 10:56 a.m.: "Just checking in with you. Want to talk to you about something. Call me when you can. Thank you." Bradee had received two text messages and two missed calls from me. "I knew something was up," she said later.

Something was up indeed. I had been taking Coumadin since 1997, when doctors discovered my blood-clotting deficiency. It's a genetic disorder known as Factor V Leiden, which is a mutation of the clotting factors, one that can cause dangerous, abnormal blood clots. My mother and grandmother also had the deficiency.

In 1997, while we were living in Jacksonville, Florida, I spent three days in St. Vincent Hospital with a blood clot in one of my legs. The pain was tremendous. The clot soon broke off and went through my heart and into my lungs. If it had lodged in my heart, Carol probably would be a widow today. That was a really sensitive time. And it was Christmastime, for goodness sake. Not a good time to be in a hospital. But Carol made it special, as usual, by cooking her traditional Christmas supper and bringing it to the hospital for the family and me to enjoy.

I thought I was out of the woods for good. It had been nearly twenty years since that first blood clot, and I had been on Coumadin the whole time. What could go wrong?

Coumadin can fail. That's what can go wrong. My INR—International Normalized Ratio, a lab measurement used to determine the effects of anticoagulants such as Coumadin—is supposed to be between three and four. For me, any measurement below three puts me at risk for blood clots. If I'd made it to Cumming that day, I would have taken time to get my INR checked. I normally had it checked once a month, and I was a little overdue. My INR obviously had fallen below three.

After she got one of my messages, Bradee wanted to rush home to get me. The charge nurse said, no, you need to call an ambulance. So Bradee found Carol and the two of them headed home. They called 911 on the way.

"An ambulance is coming to get you. Don't be alarmed," Bradee told me by phone.

My response was that of a typical macho male who played basketball and football in high school and college, who worked out to stay in shape, who was used to running up and down basketball courts and football fields, blowing a whistle. "I'm not getting in an ambulance," I told her. "I called you to check me out. I didn't call you to call an ambulance."

Bradee was the first to diagnose the problem. EMTs who answered the 911 call didn't think the problem was serious. I had walked to the ambulance just fine; I could hold out my arms just fine. But Bradee didn't think I looked normal.

"He has had a stroke," she told the EMTs.

"No, I don't think so," one of them spoke up.

"Are you going to use your siren?" Bradee demanded. "We need to get him there if there is any chance of using this medicine."

The medicine she referred to is called TPA—an abbreviation for tissue plasminogen activator. If administered soon enough, say, within the first four hours of a stroke, TPA can break up a clot before it has a chance to damage the brain. But it doesn't work for everybody. I couldn't take the medicine because I was on Coumadin. Taking a strong clot-buster like TPA was too risky for someone on a blood thinner.

The ambulance arrived at the emergency room, and I was taken to the first room available. Doctors and nurses were there to make general observations and to check blood pressure and vital signs. Then they wanted to give me an MRI, which stands for Magnetic Resonance Imaging. It means being put into a narrow tube, especially small for a big man like me, and enduring loud sounds. Being claustrophobic, I told them I was feeling a lot better.

"No," they said, "we need to find out."

"OK," I said, "y'all give me some drugs and I'll do it." They gave me Ativan, which made me loopy but also less agitated about getting screamed at by a machine shaped like a huge cigar butt.

I exited the MRI machine, and they knew for certain: I had suffered a stroke. My left arm had started to draw up while I was in the emergency room. Not a good sign.

Bradee said I was totally zonked after the MRI. Then a physician's assistant announced the verdict: "Yep," he said, "what I thought. He has had a stroke."

"Like it was no big deal," Bradee said later. "I was flabbergasted. No sympathy, no empathy, no nothing when he told us that news. That's my *Dad*!"

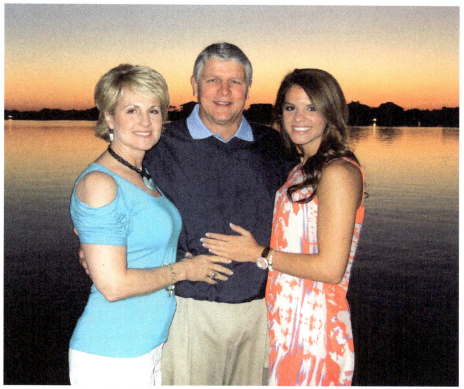

L to R: Carol Burrell, Steve and daughter Bradee.

I was taken to ICU, a perfect place for me because Bradee works in ICU. She was there to check on me every day, and she knew about stroke victims because she had seen plenty of them in her four years in ICU.

As it turned out, nothing could've been done that wasn't done. I couldn't take the TPA; the doctors and nurses were attentive; they did everything they could do. In fact, I couldn't have gotten better care. But, let me tell you, it was an emotional time. Bradee and Carol broke down and cried. I cried. If you looked at me and said "Watermelon," I'd start crying. My pastor, Dr. Tom Smiley, came to see me in ICU. I cried. Bill Risinger came to see me. I cried. Some of my football friends came to see me; others called. I got emotional. Dr. Jerry Gill of Lakewood visited every day which was an inspiration.

My officiating crew was going to be at the Georgia Dome for the big game, and I would not be there. Last year, the crew had used the slogan "teamwork makes the dream work" as we worked hard to be selected for one of the State Championship games and it also became an encouragement for me as I was challenged to work hard to improve. The next day, I listened to the Lakewood concert online. That was emotional, too, but it felt good to hear it.

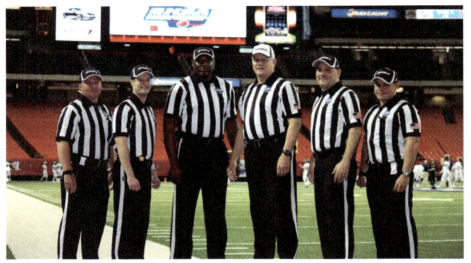

Steve with his Lanier Football Officials Association crew.
L to R: Mark Staton, Brian Kovach, Bo Hairston,
Steve, Chris Schmus, John Heath.

Effects of the stroke were in full force once I reached ICU. I had gotten into the MRI machine just fine. But now, I couldn't move my left side at all. My left leg and my left arm just hung there, practically lifeless.

But staff members at the medical center aren't there to feel sorry for you. They're there to help you get better. So, on my very first day in ICU, believe it or not, one of the inpatient therapists, Lynn Mackes, came in and said, "It's time for therapy."

Therapy? I couldn't even get out of bed. My therapy that day was to sit up, get out of bed and into a chair. With a walker and a little help, I did it. It wasn't pretty, but I did it.

The second day, Lynn fetched me a walker and walked with me down the hall for quite a distance. Again, it wasn't pretty. I shuffled along, trying to drag my left leg. And she made me use my left arm sometimes. If I didn't, she told me to do it again.

I was still pretty emotional, and although my facial droop had worsened, I had to start speech therapy. The therapist wanted me to overemphasize my words and vowels: *ooh, eeh, ah*, moving my mouth more noticeably as I spoke.

I started calling Lynn the Witch Doctor, and she called me Big Dog. When she came in one day, I told her to listen to my song: "I told the Witch Doctor, I fell in love with you. … And then the Witch Doctor, he told me what to do. He told me, 'Ooh, eeh, ooh, ah, ah, ting, tang, walla, walla, bing bang.'" They were very bad lyrics from "Witch Doctor," a song from the late fifties.

I'm not sure Lynn was impressed.

Care in ICU was excellent, and everybody was telling me I was doing well. The doctors tried to encourage me. But their encouragement didn't make me feel a whole lot better. I could move only my little finger on my left hand. But the Witch Doctor kept on pushing, and Bradee made videos so I could see how bad I was, or how good I was, however you want to look at it.

After four nights in ICU, I was sent to a regular room for a few days. From there, my destiny was inpatient rehab, but only after I met certain requirements. For starters, I had to be able to walk. No cane, no walker, no anything. I had to walk with "no compensation," as my therapist, John Higgins, put it. And I did it.

A doctor put me on Prozac, which helped get my emotions under control. I eventually got better, which means I didn't cry as much. I also was prescribed Trazodone, which helps me sleep and serves as an antidepressant, and Eliquis, which takes the place of Coumadin and requires no INR checks.

I was making progress. On December 12th, I had walked one hundred feet with a walker. On the 13th, I walked one hundred thirty feet with a walker. On the 14th, I got up without having to put a hand on a walker. I also took two hundred ninety steps that day. On the 15th, I walked without a walker. We weren't concentrating on distance at that point. We were focused on functionality. It I took one step, it had better be perfect, or at least as good as I could make it.

There was a time when little therapy was given and stroke patients were told, "You won't use that hand or that leg like you used to." But now, the first day at our medical center, patients start therapy. "The sooner you get those parts moving," Bradee said, "the quicker the recovery time."

In layman's language, therapy teaches the stroke patient's brain to fire nerves so that his arms and legs will move. To do that, he must use them. I would say to myself, "I know I can move my arm." But the part of the brain that tells the muscle to move is now impaired. Therapy helps create paths around the affected areas of the brain.

In rehab, I had my crying under control, but I got angry. I would talk to my leg: "Come on, let's go." I'd talk to my arm and hand. Anger helped sometimes because it encouraged me to go on. I already knew how the progression would play out. My leg would come back first, doctors said, and then my arm from my shoulder down to my hand. The last things I'll be able to do are the small, delicate tasks using my fingers.

Everybody's stoke is different. Doctors can't promise a stroke victim when they will get better. For some people, it's three months; for some, six months; for others, a few years. But if I put in the work, Bradee and the doctors assured me, I will see positive results.

Guess where I was on Christmas Day. Yes, as Yogi Berra famously said, "It was déjà vu, all over again." Just as it was in 1997, I spent Christmas Eve and Christmas Day of 2016 in the hospital. That was tough. But, again, my thoughtful wife made Christmas breakfast and Christmas dinner, and our family gathered in a conference room to enjoy being with each other. My mother was also there. Then we went to a Christmas concert in the hospital chapel. That was great. At least we had a semblance of a real Christmas.

On December 30th—twenty-three days after a stroke changed my life—I walked out of the hospital. But therapy continues. It continues at a rehab center not far from the hospital. During the first three months, friends and family hauled me around, from home to rehab and then back home. Therapy also continued at home. Bradee has been wonderful in helping me negotiate stairs, in walking, in sitting down correctly, in working out in our gym, in opening a carton of yogurt. "You can do it, Dad," she said after I asked her one day to open my yogurt. "You can do it." And I did.

I walk to the mail box every day. I can take a shower; I can put on my clothes, although I can't tie my shoes or don those darn compression socks yet without help.

On February 5th, I sang in the church choir for the first time since early December. My voice may not have been as strong as it once was, but it's improving every day. On Sunday, March 5th, I felt like I was sixteen again. I drove to church. I can't drive long distances now; I can't drive at night or in congested traffic. But I can drive short distances.

What does the future hold for me? I'm not sure. My original goal was to have recovered completely in three months. As this piece is written, in March of 2017, it has been three months. I have made progress, for sure, but I have not completely recovered. My enunciation has come back well; I do not slur my words anymore. I am walking better all the time. But the doctors were correct when they said my hand, my fingers, would be the last to recover. Progress, it seems, is awfully slow.

Going back to church and studying the Word have helped keep me going. Two verses of Scripture have been especially helpful. One is Philippians 4:13: "I can do all things through Christ who strengthens me." The other is Psalms 50:15: "And call on Me in the day of trouble; I will deliver you, and you will honor Me."

I can't say enough about the great support I've received from my family and friends. I knew I had a lot of friends—I'm a rather gregarious fellow—but I didn't know I had so many friends! I try not to feel sorry for myself. At first, I asked myself, "Why did this have to happen to me?" Later, I realized, "Why not me? "

I've set goals. My overall goal, of course, is to recover. But I also have specific goals. First, in mid-April, about a month from the time of this writing, Carol and I are scheduled to visit our son, Lee, who works and lives in Columbus, Ohio. From there, we'll go on to Chicago, where Carol has a business meeting and where we plan to attend the popular play "Hamilton." My next goal comes in June, when Carol and I will take a two-week trip to France. We're meeting friends there and taking a riverboat cruise. As you might imagine, there'll be a lot of walking, too, and I want to be ready. Doctors told me I would need more rest—make that *naps*—and they were right. At first, it was a four-or five-hour nap after rehab; now it's only an hour or so.

My Number Three goal, and the most important, is to be back on the football field officiating football games in September. I have officiated games in Florida and Georgia for twenty-six years, and I'm not ready to stop now. But, I must be realistic. If I don't make that September goal, I can't afford to sit back and moan. I need substitute goals. For instance, if I can't officiate on the field as a referee, I can run the game clock or mentor other officials and help teach the rules of the game, or something like that. I still want to be involved. It might be discouraging if I can't be one of the field officials, but it won't be catastrophic because there are other things I can do.

Mantra of the officiating crew, and reminder to Steve while in the hospital.

In the meantime, I don't expect to return to work. For thirty-eight years, I have been a territory sales representative for Johns Manville, but I had planned on retiring at the end of 2016. My stroke just advanced that date a bit.

But I do plan to stay active doing something. I'm trimmer now—I've lost over twenty-five pounds since my stroke. Carol likes that, but my clothes don't fit very well now.

I know this: <u>God has a plan for me</u>! For one thing, I expect to have a new testimony. I will be able to share with other people on how I got through this, how important it is to have a faith base, how important it is to have a church to support you. I hope to testify to people who might not understand the tremendous power of God.

The first Sunday I was back in the Lakewood choir after my stroke, our special was "The Church Triumphant," another Gaither favorite.

"Let the anthems ring out, songs of victory swell
For the church triumphant, is alive and well."

I praise God for those lyrics, that the church is alive and well. And I praise Him also that I am alive and well. Not as well as I hope to be one day. But I'm working on it. I'm working hard on it, and by the grace of God I'll get there!

So check with me again in a few months.

Yolanda Giddens story

(As told by Yolanda Giddens and daughter Debra Brown)

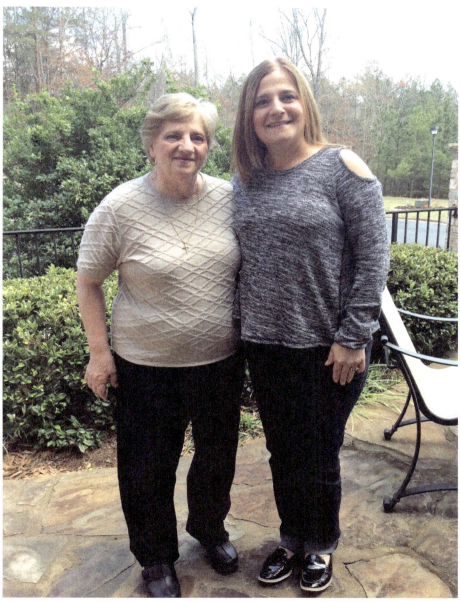

Yolanda Giddens and daughter Debra Brown

L ONG BEFORE I WAS A nurse's assistant in Statesboro Georgia, I was a practicing nurse in the city where I was born, Naples, Italy. As a child during World War II, I had long awaited liberation from the axis powers, and, as a result, I always had a fondness for American servicemen. Little did I know, I would later marry one. He was a US sailor named Joe Giddens. He was stationed in Naples, and after a whirlwind courtship, he enticed me to be his wife by asking if I would like a tour of the USS Shangri-La, a US warship harbored in the local port. The enticement worked, and we were subsequently married in Italy, and soon thereafter, our son, Joe Jr., was born. Soon after his birth, we embarked on Joe's next assignment, which was on the island of Bermuda. I said goodbye to my family and homeland, and hello to being the wife of a US sailor.

The most meaningful thing that occurred on the beautiful British isle of Bermuda was the birth of our second child, a daughter we named Debra. I never got to fully experience Bermuda while we were there. I was too busy raising two children, and besides, a tour of the island would have had to occur on a moped as we had sold our car. After three years, we were deployed to Charleston, South Carolina, where I had my first experience living with Americans in the continental United States and the confusion of the southern American accent. For the longest time, I didn't realize 'uwana' was southern for 'Do you want to…? '

From there, it was on to the Naval air station in Jacksonville, Florida, where our third child was born, a daughter we named Alma. That was our last Naval assignment, and upon Joe's retirement from the Navy, we settled into his hometown of Statesboro, Georgia. My mother and dad and eight siblings never seemed so far away.

After three moves and three children, and being an Italian now living in the deep south of the United States, I had the challenge of going from speaking Italian to learning English as the Brits spoke in Bermuda, to learning American English, complete with a deep southern drawl.

I also had my first experience learning to cook grits. I had always assumed grits was a variation of rice, which we enjoyed back in Italy virtually every day. Rice and eggs, anyone?

Such was my transition from Naples, Italy to south Georgia.

Once we were settled in Statesboro, I was eventually able to continue my nursing career. I initially took a job in the hospital in Claxton, Georgia, a small town some twenty miles from Statesboro. After 10 years commuting between Claxton and Statesboro, I then took a job as a nursing assistant at the hospital in Statesboro where I continued to work, mostly in pediatrics and later geriatrics... until that night.

My three children were now adults with families of their own, though I had lost my youngest daughter, Alma, to cancer at the age of 42. I could not imagine a worse experience in my lifetime.

I was now divorced and enjoying my life as a single mother and grandmother, and my work as a nursing assistant at East Georgia Medical Center. It was after a shift at the hospital one Sunday this past January that I arrived home to settle into an evening of a quiet dinner and some television. There was a special on TV about Dr. Martin Luther King, Jr. which I was enjoying until I fell asleep on the sofa.

Around midnight, I woke up to go to the bathroom. Getting up, however, I discovered I could not move my left leg and had minimal support from my left arm. Without a thought about what this might mean medically, I instinctively forced myself up to go to the bathroom. As I struggled, my medical background began to kick in and concluded I was experiencing a stroke.

In the midst of it all, I flashed back to the previous November when I had gone to the doctor complaining of a severe pain in my legs. I found myself wondering if that was related to what I was now experiencing.

Though the hour was late, I called my son, Joe Jr. He immediately came over and drove me to the hospital. The emergency room doctors confirmed my worst fear. I was analyzed, diagnosed, and treated in the emergency room, and then admitted to the hospital for additional treatment and therapy.

Joe Jr. called his sister who lived in Gainesville Georgia, some five hours away, to give her the bad news. It was 2 AM. "No one", said daughter Debra Brown, "calls you to share good news at 2 o'clock in the morning." She hastily made arrangements for the 5 Hour drive to Statesboro.

I had left the hospital earlier that day as an employee, and returned later that night as a patient.

Though bedridden by the stroke, I was able to manage the basics of my existence while in the hospital. I was able to get up and go to the bathroom on my own, but after three days, during one such trip, my left leg would no longer support me. The full effects of my stroke was still assaulting my body up to three days later. Up until then my most difficult challenge was my inability to move my left arm or use my left hand. Now I was confronted with the challenge of being able to move.

I wasn't sure if my stroke was getting better or getting worse?

After a week of treatment and therapy in the hospital in Statesboro, my daughter and son and I made a decision. We agreed that I might receive better care if I were transferred to the hospital in Gainesville, some five hours away but the home of my daughter. I would be going to one of the leading medical centers in the country for stroke-related issues, and I would be near my daughter, Debra.

We navigated our way through the hospital and insurance red tape and bureaucracy, and after nine days, I was transferred to the rehab unit in the Northeast Georgia Medical Center in Gainesville, Georgia. Their initial diagnosis concluded that the major challenges I faced were the rehabilitation of my left arm and hand, and to a lesser degree, my left leg. That diagnosis put me in the rehabilitative care of a therapist named Charlie, a delightful young woman who launched into my therapy with a series of exercises designed to help me regain the use of my left arm and hand.

When you spend a month in the hospital, you have a lot of quiet time to ponder how all of this happened. There were times when I could not avoid the question, 'Why me?' Was I enjoying my life too much? Was I being punished for some reason? Was this God's way of preparing me for something bigger in my life? I knew Debra was prepared to take me into her home, but she and her husband have a family to take care of. And I had a job to return to and a home that was awaiting my return. I was eager to put this behind me and get on with my life, yet no doctor would tell me how long I would have to endure this, or if I faced the prospects of a second stroke. Too much time to think and too many questions.

After two weeks of therapy in Gainesville, I was discharged from my second hospital within a month, then off to live with my daughter, Debra, and continue my therapy on an outpatient basis.

She had either read a book on tough love, or was getting even for something that must've happened in her childhood, because once in her home, I found myself on the floor with her doing sit-ups and push-ups and all sorts of other exercises . And I had outpatient therapy sessions to attend. In reality, she was not only the perfect hostess, but the perfect coach and supervisor.

Now, though I am enjoying my time with my daughter and her beautiful family, it is time for me to return to my home in Statesboro, and the job I love. I am enjoying my exercises and therapy sessions, but I still have some work to do. I walk with the best of them, but continue to experience stiffness in my hand... not the best way to return to a nursing job.

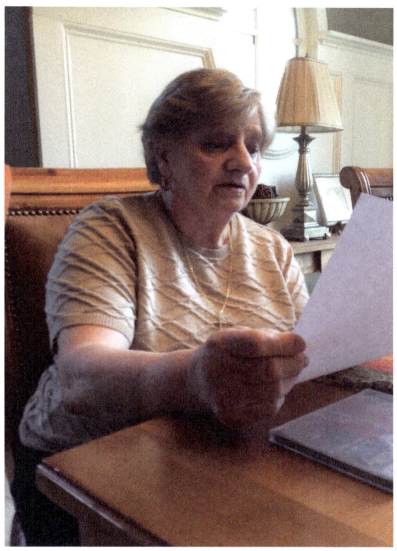

Me, pondering my future.

It is my left hand that currently stands between me and my return to a nursing career and to the life of a fully functioning human being.

I am looking forward to the day.

Frederick Blair story

(As told by Frederick Blair)

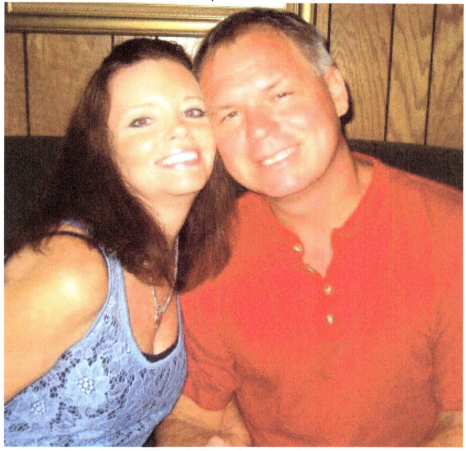

Michelle and Frederick

MY LIFE WAS SIMPLE... FAMILY, carpentry, construction, hunting, and fishing. No complications, no drama, nothing to keep me up at night, unless I chose to do so. I had a place on the lake. I could work when I wanted. Our two daughters were grown and developing lives of their own. It was just me and my wife, Michelle, at home and enjoying life. The year 2016 did its dead level best to change all of that.

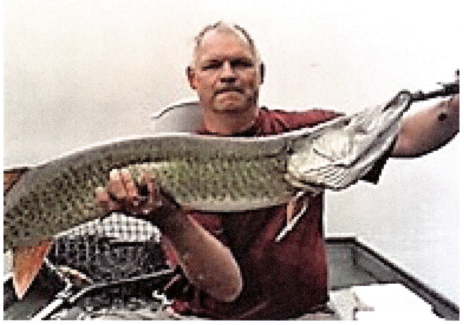

Frederick and trophy.

My first indication of what 2016 held in store for me was when in March of that year, my wife totaled her car. Fortunately, she was not seriously injured, but an automobile accident is never fun. I jokingly told Michelle her accident was probably an omen of things to come. Little did I know just how prophetic I would be. Things continued to go downhill from there.

A little more than a month later, that prophecy proved itself to be correct once again. My working partner and boss, someone with whom I had enjoyed a 16 year personal and professional relationship, ended his life. He had endured bouts of depression and alcoholism over the years, but we had hoped those days were behind him. They were not.

His death took a toll on me, both personally and professionally. I had to find a way to soldier on. It is hard to work with someone side-by-side for 16 years and not be affected by his loss.

As the year unfolded, so did the calamities.

As if one automobile accident was not enough, it was my daughter, Kayla's, turn. Barely a month after my partner's death, like Michelle, she totaled her car. And like Michelle, she was fortunate she avoided serious injury. As we were recovering from Michelle and Kayla's accidents, I could not help wonder what would be next. I would soon find out.

My father had been struggling with his health for some time. In August of that year, he passed away. His death further complicated the year as I was left with the emotional issues of losing my father, plus the issues of handling his estate.

Following my father's death, I suffered a cold and persistent cough that I was unable to shake. For more than two months, I was on a steady diet of cold medicines and cough syrup. During that time, I suspected my unshakable cold was the latest, and hopefully the last, incident in a series of events that marked a year I would just as soon forget. It was not.

On December 12, I embarked on a deer hunting expedition, using a portable tree stand that would give me the ability to shimmy up a tree and wait for the unsuspecting game. It was a device I had used many times, and was considered highly reliable.

On this occasion, I was in the woods adjacent to my house and picked out a tree I thought would serve as the perfect spot. After climbing about 15 feet up the tree I had selected, I noticed a pen was missing from the harness that secured the device to the tree. I decided to descend back to the ground to repair the device. I believed my arm strength would substitute for the harness temporarily to allow me to hold on to the tree as I descended back down to the ground. I was wrong.

In a matter of seconds, I fell to the ground and was temporarily knocked unconscious. I recall waking to find myself sprawled on the ground on my back and my left leg awkwardly pushed out to one side. The pain was indescribable. As I attempted to regain my composure I also attempted to bring my left leg back underneath my body, but it refused to move. I knew then that I was in trouble. I was in the middle of the woods, in immense pain, and unable to move.

Fortunately, I had my cell phone with me and was able to call Michelle who was on her way to a school Christmas party. I briefly described what had happened and asked her to call our neighbor to ask him if he could come to my rescue. Thankfully, he did.

As I waited, I began to ponder the steady diet of call medication I had been taking. I wondered if my judgment or my physical abilities had been hampered by the effects of that medication. I shall never know.

My neighbor drove his pontoon boat over close to where I had fallen. He was able to locate me and immediately called 911. He then waited with me as the EMS crew eventually navigated their way through the woods to where I was located. Once they found our location using GPS technology, they then had the issue of getting me back to their vehicle on a stretcher and transporting me to the hospital. Finally, two hours after that fateful fall, I found myself lying in the emergency room at Northeast Georgia Medical Center.

Michelle never made it to her Christmas party. She returned home after receiving my call only to learn that I was already being transported to the emergency room, where she then proceeded to meet me.

The ER doctors quickly ruled out my initial assumption that I had broken my leg from the fall. They concluded instead the problem was with my back. The backbone and vertebrae are categorized into six sections or regions. One of those is called the Lumbar region and one of those is the Thoracic region. X-rays revealed that the L1 (Lumbar one) vertebrae had suffered a burst fracture, and the L2 had been dislocated, as was the T11 (Thoracic 11) and T12 vertebrae. Additionally I suffered spinal cord damage which resulted in a temporary paralysis of my legs and was the biggest challenge I would face in my recovery.

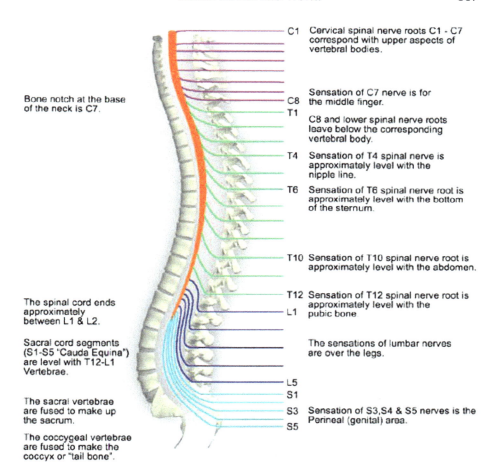

Bone notch at the base of the neck is C7.

The spinal cord ends approximately between L1 & L2.

Sacral cord segments (S1-S5 "Cauda Equina") are level with T12-L1 Vertebrae.

The sacral vertebrae are fused to make up the sacrum.

The coccygeal vertebrae are fused to make the coccyx or "tail bone".

C1 — Cervical spinal nerve roots C1 - C7 correspond with upper aspects of vertebral bodies.

C8 / T1 — Sensation of C7 nerve is for the middle finger.

C8 and lower spinal nerve roots leave below the corresponding vertebral body.

T4 — Sensation of T4 spinal nerve is approximately level with the nipple line.

T6 — Sensation of T6 spinal nerve root is approximately level with the bottom of the sternum.

T10 — Sensation of T10 spinal nerve root is approximately level with the abdomen.

T12 / L1 — Sensation of T12 spinal nerve root is approximately level with the pubic bone.

The sensations of lumbar nerves are over the legs.

L5 / S1

S3 / S5 — Sensation of S3, S4 & S5 nerves is the Perineal (genital) area.

I was told I would require a series of three surgical procedures. The first would be to take a bone from my rib cage and mold it into a brace to provide support to my injured spinal column. The second would be to insert the brace into my back as a support for my damaged vertebrae and spinal cord. The third, which would occur after my back had properly healed ,would be to remove the brace they had inserted from my back.

With the harshest degree of sarcasm I could muster, I thought, What better way to end an eventful 2016!

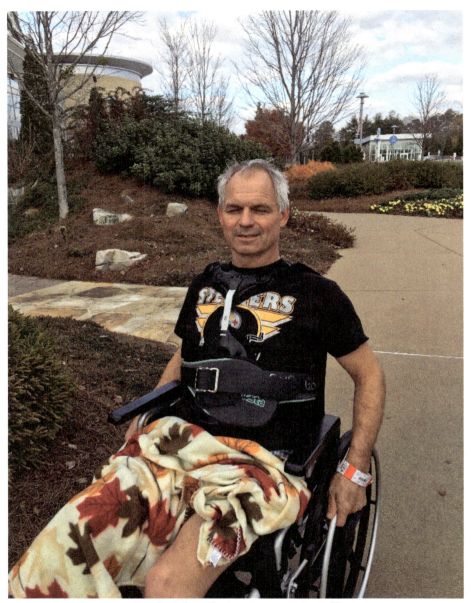

Frederick, relaxing in easy chair ⊠

After the first two surgeries and five days in the intensive care unit, I was transferred to the rehabilitation unit of the hospital to begin therapy for my paralysis. I was a fish out of water from the very beginning. There were no other patients on the unit who were recovering from a back injury. They all seemed to be stroke patients and the unit seemed to be set up to accommodate strokes, not back injuries. They didn't seem to know what to do with me.

Additionally, I was completely encumbered by a brace that extended from my waist to my chest, designed to keep me immobile while my back healed. At the time, I was much less concerned about my therapy and more concerned about my ability to go to the bathroom when I wanted. My every move was completely controlled by a medical staff that appeared not to be accustomed to dealing with a back patient. A giant pulley device, managed by the nurses, controlled my entry and exit from my bed. Talk about a loss of control.

The therapy staff seemed equally unsure about how to deal with my circumstance. This was a group accustomed to dealing with stroke patients, and though I was not a stroke patient, I was treated like one. Being asked to stand when I was completely immobilized by a back brace was the equivalent of asking a mummy to walk. They had a protocol to follow, and even though I did not fit the profile of their other patients, I was asked to adhere to that protocol. I'm sure I was not their favorite patient.

We eventually settled into a regimen that was more suited to my predicament and I actually began to make progress with my standing and walking.

I was discharged from the hospital on January 6th, almost a month after my accident, and continued my therapy on an outpatient basis. Once again, I had to sort out the differences of my situation with a new therapy staff. We eventually experienced progress in repeated sessions which continued for another two months. I later navigated my way to a series of aquatic therapy treatments in the pool, where I experienced my most significant progress.

In retrospect, there were many parallels between my predicament and those of a stroke patient. I had the challenges of relearning to stand and walk and the challenges of regaining strength in my legs. One major difference, however, was going through this process all while allowing my back to heal from major surgery. In the spring time I would also face the additional challenge of yet an additional surgery to remove the support brackets from my damaged back.

In the end, I quit quibbling with the therapy staff about the differences between a patient who had suffered a broken back as compared to a patient who had suffered a stroke. The similarities were much greater than the differences and the gains from their exercises were equally valuable. Additionally, I benefited greatly from my interactions with many of the stroke patients who were enduring similar symptoms and on a recovery path such as mine.

The year 2017 was on track to be much better than the preceding year. For that I am eternally grateful, and though I wouldn't wish my predicament on my most evil enemy, I actually began to experience some degree of inspiration from the process. I was certainly more appreciative of my wife and two daughters, and also found myself reaching out to those around me and expressing my appreciation for them.

My life was once again becoming simple. Only this time, with more appreciation and with more of a human touch.

Welcome 2017!

* * * *

You might surmise, both from the stories cited above and general perception, that the majority of stroke survivors are male. Surprisingly, the reality seems to be the opposite. According to several statistics, the majority of stroke survivors are surprisingly female. According to stroke.org, over 50% of stroke victims are female.

Indicators suggest that strokes are highly indiscriminate in who they strike and at what age. That was the scariest notion of my research. It seems that all of us, regardless of health, diet, and other factors, are prospects for this terrible malady. Something has to change. The fraternity is growing. And our progress is mixed in restricting the number of people that become part of that fraternity.

Fortunately, there are people and organizations that are hot on the trail. The people at the National Stroke Association, (www.stroke.org) are working diligently to find the answers in the prevention and recovery of strokes. Other organizations, such as the American Heart Association and the National Center for Disease Control also are doing their parts. We applaud their efforts and look forward to doing our part. The answers cannot come soon enough.

At a minimum, we must band together. Whether 4 of us or 4 million of us, only we know our stories. Only we know the journey. Stroke groups are popping up all over the country. That is not good news given the unwanted growth of this phenomenon, but it is good news for the benefit of stroke survivors and their caregivers.

During my recovery, the Northeast Georgia stroke group was formed, and I was fortunate enough to be a part of that formation. Stroke survivors, their caregivers, and their therapists all had something in common to share. How do we better detect this malady? How do we achieve that detection faster, and provide a more effective recovery?

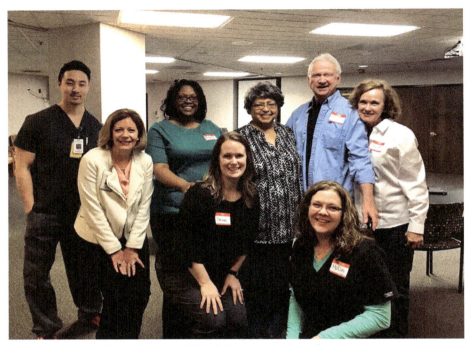

Initial meeting. North East Georgia stroke group.

The fraternity I had found myself in now had a purpose and a reason to get together and discuss. North East Georgia had joined the many other stroke groups around the country to do its part in dealing with the effects of this dreaded illness.

CHAPTER 9
Death, Debilitation, or Recovery

L IKE POLIO, CANCER AND AIDS, the term 'stroke' is one of those that many equate with death or some type of debilitation. There is another outcome. One that is seldom mentioned but fortunately, is very achievable. And that is achieving a complete recovery. With the exception of only those who experience the most extreme variation of a stroke, it comes down to a matter of work. For some, the work required is longer and harder, but it remains a matter of work. The medical community knows it. And most who have survived a stroke know it. Much of the rest of the country, however, has yet to grasp that reality. It is our job to educate them.

Everyone knows of someone that did not survive a stroke. My father is a prime example. Likewise, everyone knows of someone who suffered some form of disability from a stroke. Residing in the shadows, however, many know of someone who not only survived a stroke, but has resumed a normal, healthy lifestyle. It is those that we need to give more attention. It is those that we need to celebrate.

If you are a stroke survivor and fortunate enough to have gotten past the first outcome of death from a stroke, then chances are good you are also fortunate enough to choose between the second or the third option. After two days in the hospital following my stroke, I realized that I had a chance to fully recover… if I was willing to put in the work. Fortunately, most other stroke survivors have the same attitude.

After spending two days feeling sorry for myself and being angry at my circumstances, I decided the third outcome was the one I would pursue. I wanted to achieve a complete recovery, and given the combination of medical technology and therapeutic resources, I knew it was possible.

My goal was a complete recovery but I quickly realized that achieving that goal was contingent on me working harder than anything I have ever done in my life. It is like that obese person determined to lose hundred pounds. If I was willing to dedicate myself to the work and the lifestyle, that goal was achievable and entirely up to me.

My therapy began to take on a purpose. Rather than being a burden and an inconvenience at a time when all I wanted to do was rest, I began to see therapy as my roadmap to recovery… a series of necessary steps to achieve my objective. I suddenly found myself wanting to be the hardest working man in the hospital. If the therapist said let's do 20 reps, I would do 30. If the therapist said let's walk 50 feet, I wanted to walk 100. I viewed every step of my rehabilitation as a necessary step towards my recovery. No step was unavoidable. There were no shortcuts.

The therapy staff knew. My family knew. The majority of the other stroke survivors also knew. Though that was a revelation to me, nothing I was discovering was new information. It was common knowledge… You do the work, you get the results.

My roadmap was one of those things that was now easy to see, and easy to say, but difficult to do. The road I had embarked on was monumental. I was required to work harder than I ever had in my life at a time when my body was least capable, and the end was nowhere in sight.   But I was reminded of the saying, 'Once you start dancing with the bear, you can't stop just because you're tired.' I was embarked on a path that I could not abandon, nor did I want to.

Many choices in our lives are rather ambiguous. The black and white in our world many times comes with a touch of gray…. sort of like the song by the Grateful Dead. This is not one of those. Assuming we have cleared the first of three options… survival, the remaining two options, some form of debilitation or a complete recovery, are largely up to us. How important was it to me to regain the independence I once enjoyed? How meaningful was it to enjoy the full use of my body without compromising or compensating for certain tasks or circumstances? How important was it to be a fully functioning human being, and not have conditions or restrictions on what I can or cannot do? And how important was it to let my family and friends know, mine is not a form of debilitation, but merely a temporary inconvenience.

I have said repeatedly, this is the hardest work I've ever done. After a grueling therapy session, the last thing I wanted to do was go home and exercise. What I wanted to do was go home and sleep. My body was not prepared to do the amount of effort seemingly required to achieve the goal. 'It's all about the work,' was a handy expression, but many times, it was the last thing I wanted to do.

How much was I willing to push? How much was I willing to test the boundaries of my body's ability? Or my will? At times, not much. The body was at times unwilling, and I was uncertain if the gains being made were worth the effort.

I had to find the balance between listening to my body and pushing my body. Marathon training had taught me the tough lesson that I should pay attention to my body and not overwork, but never like this. I had never been this weak or this crippled before. I had never been this uncertain before. There were lessons I had not yet learned, and though there were many helpful sources, I had yet to find the teacher that had the answer.

If I pushed excessively, would that accelerate my recovery? If I rested, would my body simply heal on it's on? *(Boxing vs. judo)*. My doctors had opinions. My therapists had opinions. My family had opinions. But none of them had ever experienced a stroke. Ultimately, the answer was mine alone to discover, and would be found largely in the work I was willing to undertake. I felt I was in uncharted waters and ultimately I had only myself on which to rely. I knew God was with me, but I think He was saying to me, 'Ross, you've got this.'

CHAPTER 10
Ultimately, The Battle is Mine

THE WORK AND SUPPORT OF the doctors, nurses, therapists and medical staff was incredible. I would not be here if not for their expertise, professionalism, care and support they provided, especially in the earliest days of my stroke. The love and support of Jennifer and my family was and has been invaluable through my stroke and my recovery. Every step I took in my rehabilitation and my recovery was partially motivated with them in mind. The support of my friends was in every way appreciated and extremely valuable. My entire support team was exceptional. But in the darkest nights, laying in the hospital bed, and later in my own bed, exercising at 3 AM and alone with my own thoughts, I realized this is a battle only I could fight. Ultimately, I was on my own.

Most of us have family and caretakers that support us every step of the way. But family and friends cannot fight the battle. I realized that, like birth and death, this was a journey I must take by myself.

It was my first such battle. And there was no magic bullet, no quick fix, and no real roadmap to follow. Remember, *"It depends. Every case is different""*

I had witnessed family members undergo heart procedures that could have been life or death. I make another reference to my sister who survived breast cancer. I watched my parents and my oldest sister ultimately succumb to their illnesses. I even came close myself once before. But I don't remember ever being confronted face-to-face with the loneliness of such a battle. How does one prepare?

I found myself even having to work through the battle of loneliness and isolation alone. Friends can sympathize and empathize with you, even those who are fighting a similar battle, but ultimately the battle must be fought and won by myself.

I was constantly reminded of those whose battle was far worse than my own and that unlike others, I would eventually recover. I knew I would improve to regain my previous level of capability. Others could not make that claim. Some now faced a debilitating lifestyle, one less than they had once enjoyed. I found myself suddenly interested to know their story as well as tell my own. What were their survival techniques? How did they sustain themselves? How did they maintain a positive attitude in the face of a terrible situation?

The fraternity I had been initiated into was not only larger than I had anticipated, but more selective. Those that felt sorry for themselves need not apply. Ours was a fraternity that included the broadest range of maladies, but only those who embraced and courageously confronted their fight. It was a fraternity of individuals who confronted their circumstances with bravery and determination, and chose to fight, knowing it would be alone.

Like so many others, I faced a battle I would ultimately have to fight by myself, but I yearned to know the story of those who were engaged in similar battles. I wanted to learn their techniques, their attitude, their source of their bravery, in hopes that some of that may rub off on me.

This is without question not only the toughest battle I have had to fight, but the loneliest. I was not the first, nor will I be the last. There is a sign over a flight school which reads, "Learn from the lessons of others. You will not survive to learn them all by yourself." I wanted to learn the lessons of others… their battles, their desolate journeys.

Many nights at 3 AM, with nothing to disturb me but the nurses coming in at various times of the night to check on me, I reflected on just what had happened and what my future held. I remained steadfastly confident of the destination, but completely uncertain of the journey. How long would it take? Just how much work would it be? I had questions about what was in store for me unlike any before, and was eager to learn from those that preceded me.

If there was ever a time for soul-searching in my life, this was it. I had been thrown a giant curveball which upended my entire life. Whatever plans I had for myself had to be reassessed. Whatever legacy and memories I was to leave for my grandchildren had to be re-thought. Whatever purpose my life was to serve had to be re-examined.

My faith in God was undying, and I knew He was there to ensure I reached my destination. With that knowledge however, I felt He had given me this challenge in preparation for what they ever awaited me. If God places events in your life to shape your destination, was this placed in my life to serve a purpose? Was there a way my circumstance could serve a meaningful purpose for others? Was there a way for me to turn this giant lemon into lemonade? Was that now my challenge?

I found myself increasingly empathetic and curious about the lives of others who have special needs of some sort. I was in the midst of writing a story about a woman who had suffered a boating accident and came close to losing her legs. She spent years going through rehabilitation and was required to relearn how to walk. I remember her describing the exhaustion of walking 500 feet. I could now relate in ways that I could have never before.

I found myself reaching out to other stroke patients, as well as others who were experiencing stroke like symptoms to learn their stories. How were they coping?

What does one do when they do not have the means or circumstances to endure the loss of their work or income? The medical bills? The dependence on others? What does one do when they do not have the support team, the group of caregivers, there to assist them as they undergo their recovery? Theirs is a battle which, before this happened to me, I would have been sympathetic to, but not truly understanding of.

There is a segment of the population who face those battles every day while the rest of the world goes about their business. I was now a part of that population, even though only temporarily, and had to be prepared. Everyone who lives in that world receives varying degrees of love, support and assistance, but the battles they face are ultimately theirs as the battle I faced was ultimately mine. Much of that preparation was physical, but so much more was emotional and spiritual.

During my days in the hospital, I was visited by individuals that represented various organizations that provided support to stroke survivors. But the most striking visit I received was not from a victim of a stroke, but an automobile accident. His name was Scotty Hunt and he and his mother had written a book entitled "Why Scotty?" His story was that of a promising college athlete whose life was turned completely upside down when the vehicle in which he was riding was in a horrific accident.

Though due to circumstances of a different making, he suffered many symptoms that stroke victims suffer. Accompanied by his mother, he shared his story. After months of recovery and rehabilitation, he devoted his life to helping others who had experienced similar circumstances. His is one whose life was not only changed. His entire purpose was changed.

Scotty was an inspiration to me, yet underscored the isolated nature of my recovery. As I read his book, I was reminded of the loneliness of the vigil. His was a moving story that gave me strength and preparation for my own lonely vigil.

Another source of inspiration was a book written by the former New England Patriots linebacker, Tedy Bruschi. Given my affinity for the New England Patriots, I was particularly interested in his story, as he suffered his stroke at the age of 31, and yet managed to return once again to play professional football, the sport he loved so well. His book, co-authored by the Boston Globe sports columnist, Michael Holly, was entitled "Never Give Up." His story also was one of fighting a lonely but successful battle of recovery, leading to his return to professional football.

The stories of those around me were equally inspiring, yet equally desolate in their battle. Steve Burrell, Frederick Blair, Yolanda Giddens and the many others who shared their stories, spoke of battles only they could fight. Though their stories gave me words of inspiration, they also remind me of the loneliness of the journey that confronts each of us.

I did not choose the fraternity I had joined. I did not choose the lonely journey that was thrust upon me. But I had slowly come to terms with what lay before me. With the love and support of my family, friends and healthcare professionals that were critical to my recovery, much the way a marathon runner ventures off on a long run, I had begun.

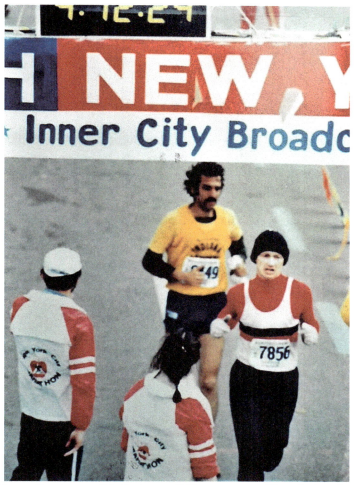

Me, earlier in my life facing a different type of lonely battle…
my first New York Marathon in 30 degree temperatures.

I came to conclude ours is not a journey to be looked upon with pity or sorrow, but one of inspiration. It is one we must travel alone, knowing God will be watching over us, and our family and loved ones will be waiting for us at the end.

Once I concluded this is a battle that no one else could fight but me, I was faced with the stark realization of my choice. I could either sit (or lay, as the current circumstance dictated) passively and succumb to the battle, or face the battle head-on and ultimately conquer the beast.

The realization of my isolation, the realization that no one else could fight the battle but me, increased my sense of determination. There was really no choice in the matter. I would not be defeated by my circumstances, especially when I had the medical odds in my favor. Less than 20% of the people who suffer strokes die. Less than 40% experience any form of lasting debilitation. That meant over 60% of stroke survivors were given the opportunity to experience a full recovery. Did I want to be a part of the first two categories? One of those who experienced death or debilitation? Absolutely not.

One question that has continually eluded me through this journey, however, and does so to this day, is the fine line between those who do the work, those who refuse to do the work, and those who are unable to do the work. I had become highly sensitive to and wanted to know more about those who have experienced more severe strokes. For them, it may not be all about the work. The work and the attitude must be present in their efforts to recover, but we must recognize the severity of their situation and hope that medical technology can further their efforts.

The more I examined my circumstance, the more I knew my stroke was relatively mild, despite the early days of my paralysis, and I was presented the opportunity for a full recovery. Those who had suffered some form of debilitation faced a much greater battle than my own. In the larger scheme of things, mine was merely an inconvenience. A temporary interruption to my life that would provide me a new lease on life, and a new purpose.

It is those thoughts at 3 AM that ultimately led me to write this book. I am an author. I am a ghostwriter. I work with individuals to help them write their biographies, their memoirs, their stories. People share with me highly personal accounts of stories of loneliness, love, death, maladies and other events that have affected their life. Their ups, their downs, their battles, their defeats and their victories. I now had one of those events that has affected my life. I now had a story to tell. One that will not only speak for me, but hopefully for the millions of individuals whose circumstance has been equally if not far more challenging than my own. I potentially had the power to share my story in hopes that it would speak for others.

I have written a number of books in my life, many of which were written with strong conviction. But I would never write a book as personal and with the power of my convictions, as this one. I was now empowered and even more eager to take on this battle. I wanted to write not only for myself, but for the millions of individuals whose circumstances were far more challenging than my own.

My lonely battle had given me a new mission, a new sense of purpose.

So what if I couldn't write the way I did before? Before that day in December? So what if I had to rely more on my left hand? A hand that was far weaker and less nimble than it was pre-stroke? Until my right arm and hand were strong enough to resume their natural place and role in my life, my left hand would simply have to carry the burden.

My book might not be a commercial venture as much as it will be a labor of conviction. I am less interested in how many books I sell and more interested in simply sharing my story, and learning more about the fraternity of which I was now a part and the work we had to perform.

Even if we each had to do it alone.

CHAPTER 11
Declaration of Independence

THIS CHAPTER WAS ORIGINALLY INTENDED to analyze the array of medical research and new technologies that were advancing the prevention and the recovery of strokes. New technologies such as the brain imaging technology to identify the source of the stroke, and stent technology to remove the clot.

There are emerging technologies that not only assist in the recovery of strokes, but also in their prevention. When it came to medical research, I was quickly taken down into the scientific weeds, and would have to be a research scientist (which I'm not) to fully understand and appreciate the many advancements being made on behalf of the stroke phenomenon. While much of it is new and not yet mainstream to the consumer or even the medical community, emerging breakthroughs offer much to be optimistic about in our battle against strokes.

I met with a German based company, for example, named Bemer that provides a technology that facilitates the blood flow of the body, the critical factor in the health of a body and in the prevention of strokes. If the theme of this book is 'it's all about the work', their theme would be 'it's all about the flow.' They use what is referred to as PEMF (pulsed electromagnetic fields) technologies to generate blood flow, comes in the form of a completely passive mat, much like a yoga mat, that spreads out on your easy chair or sofa to lie upon and watch your body increase its blood flow as it did when you were a 20-year-old.

Bemer's goal is for all of us to be relaxing on one of their mats in the privacy of our homes for eight minutes, twice a day. The result is the regeneration of our blood flow, which proposes to significantly reduce, if not eliminate the incidence of strokes.

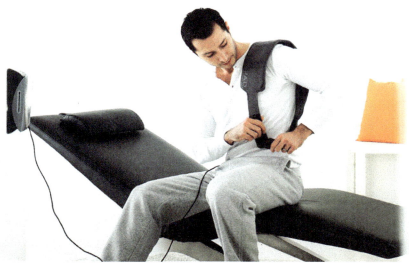

Bemer preparing to go to work.

Additionally, I met with another company, Esko Skeletal Technologies, that also employs PEMF technology to facilitate and enhance the process of walking after a stroke.

There is a company called SanBio working with the University of California San Francisco, to perfect the use of stem cells in the brain to repair damaged brain cells.

These are only the tip of the iceberg of technologies and medical science to come to enable the prevention and rehabilitation of strokes.

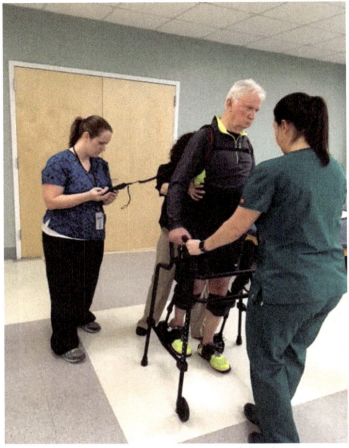

Me, with Denise and other members of the therapy team,
experimenting with new technology.

Physical therapists routinely use similar technologies such as the one
provided by the company, Bioness, to stimulate muscle movement and
promote the ability to walk. There are a number of products and advances
in medical technologies, that hopefully will someday reduce strokes to
the same category as polio and other diseases of the past... by a remedy
achieved by laying on a mat, or an inoculation or some other similar means.

New technologies seemed to be emerging every day, but those
technologies and conventional medical practices have yet to reduce the
occurrence of strokes or the ability to recover from them. So, is there hope
on the horizon?

Dr. Lee Marcus, a leading cardiologist who heads a practice entitled Preventive Cardiology of New York and serves as the Chief Medical Officer for a company called Arterial Health International, says yes. The cardiologist, a leading proponent of preventive practices, claims there is a way to identify potential strokes before they occur through adequate screening. And, he says, the technology already exists.

He explains that many doctors and individuals rely on traditional risk factors, such as blood pressure and cholesterol, to determine the risks of a potential stroke. Those risk factors, Dr. Marcus argues, often fail to identify the real source of the stroke, a blood clot embedded in our body waiting to strike. Those blood clots can only be identified through proper screening. By applying pre-screening practices, such as those used in his own practice, and the use of technologies available through companies such as Arterial Health, practitioners and individuals alike can identify the real risks and take proper measures to prevent a potential stroke. To take advantage of this technology, however, we must shift the paradigm in the healthcare community from reactive to preventive practices.

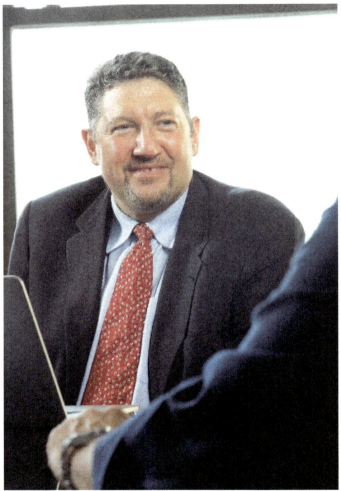

Dr. Lee Marcus, explains the virtues of preventive medicine.

I then began to wonder, are we still stuck in the mindset of fixing something that is broken rather than taking steps to prevent it from breaking? Have we come to rely too much on medical technology and conventional medical practices, and not enough on ourselves? Are we doing our part to reduce the incidence of strokes and enhance our ability to recover from them? Perhaps like the argument that we rely on police to solve social ills that should be dealt with inside the home, are we placing too much responsibility on traditional medical practices, rather than ourselves? We know there are risk factors beyond our control, such as age, race and family history, but it is equally evident that the majority of strokes are due to factors we can control, such as diet and exercise… and preventive screening.

Lester Maddox, the outspoken former governor of the state of Georgia, was once asked, how do we develop a better class of prisons in the state of Georgia? He promptly replied, 'Give me a better class of inmates, and we will have a better class of prisons.' His reply, while perhaps not politically correct, contains an element of truth. In the game of golf, new technologies and equipment now enable you to hit the ball longer, straighter, and with more consistency. Golf balls are manufactured to last longer and provide an improved ball flight. Yet, with all the innovations that have occurred over the past 50 years, golf scores remain about the same. The technology is better, yet the game is the same.

The same seems to be true with strokes. There are new technologies to enable improved prevention and better recovery techniques. Medical research has made extraordinary strides in support of predicting and preventing strokes, and in the recovery process. Yet the incidence of strokes continues to rise. Perhaps, in addition to a better class of inmates and a better class of golfers, we need a better class of healthy human beings, who take responsibility for their own health.

Daniel Keating, professor of psychology at the University of Michigan and author of "Born Anxious: The Lifelong Impact of Early Life Adversity—and How to Break the Cycle", writes 'Stress-related disorders and diseases have been on the rise in the whole population for decades, according to data from the Centers for Disease Control and Prevention, including those leading to these deaths of despair, but also to strokes, heart disease, obesity, and diabetes'. National surveys by the American Psychological Association which capture how stressed, anxious and overwhelmed we feel show a similar increasing pattern. And, according to their research, 'it shows up in our bodies, even before we get sick or start down the many roads to self-harm.'

Every first-time stroke survivor that I met or read about, who was committed to achieving a full recovery, had re-dedicated themselves to three commitments:

1) An improved heart healthy diet,
2) an exercise regimen, and
3) religiously taking their medication.

Perhaps there be a fourth action: proper screening.

As a stroke survivor and now a student of this growing phenomenon, I am hopeful of the medical technology and technologies that can be applied to strokes, but am equally hopeful that we recognize and adhere to the preventive practices and responsibilities that are ours. And if we, as stroke survivors, are a little lax in our commitment to our own responsibilities, perhaps our caregivers can remind us.

What follows is a plea to our caregivers to help us stay in line, should we incur this unfortunate malady and must travel down this lonesome road of recovery. Consider this our declaration of independence and a suggested list of reminders and guidelines, in recognition of the vital role you, the caregiver, play in achieving that recovery.

The Stroke Survivor's Declaration of Independence and Suggested Guidelines for Caregivers

Our goal is to regain our independence.

As caregivers, do everything within your power to help us attain that goal. But, be aware that your actions will either prolong our dependence on someone else, or nudge us toward the independence we so desire. It is no doubt easier and faster if you put on our socks for us, or if you tie our shoes for us, but it is infinitely better for all parties concerned, if you encourage us to do it ourselves. Be sensitive and help us with the menial tasks that we cannot yet perform on our own. But, within reason, challenge us to do more. You have a unique perspective on what we can and cannot do. Use that perspective, even to the point of irritation, to help us achieve that goal.

Our second goal is to reclaim our normalcy.

All we want is to regain the life we once lived... speak as we spoke before; smile as we smiled before; have the full motion of our arms and hands as we did before; walk as we did before. Anytime we demonstrate something less than those things, that means we have more work to do. Be gentle and loving, but remind us... help us regain our normalcy.

Monitor our therapy sessions and encourage us to do our homework.

We leave each therapy session with a series of exercises to practice at home. But when we get home, we are invariably distracted by the routines of our new life, and many times we are too tired to exercise. You have our permission to encourage, even nag us, to do our homework. Your nagging may be irritating at first, but it will benefit all of us in the long run.

Encourage us, celebrate our achievements, but never be satisfied.

Throughout our recovery, we invariably hear compliments about how well we are doing. Because so many fear being insensitive, we very seldom hear statements such as, 'That doesn't look normal', or 'I believe you can do that better.' You have our permission to tell us when you see it, or even put a mirror in front of us. Please continue to encourage us and compliment us on our progress, but urge us to do more.

Stay one step ahead of us.

As we attempt to walk, thinking we cannot go another step, please remain in front of us, urging us to take one more step, one more repetition. If we can raise our arm only to shoulder height, and you know the next step is to raise it two inches higher, urge us to do so. Remind us not to exceed our pain limit, but urge us to the next level. Determine our next milestone, and go there and wait for us. Then encourage us to catch up.

Serve as our feedback mechanism.

You observe us more than anyone else, and see our progress more than anyone else. Give us feedback. Let us know where we're making progress and what we focus on next, but likewise, let us know when our actions 'look like crap.' If we challenge your observation, put a mirror in front of us or video tape us. Give us feedback. Help us honestly and sensitively know our status, and what lies before us.

Please forgive our lack of filter.

One of the potential byproducts of having a stroke, is losing our filtering mechanism, our ability to choose our words carefully, resulting in us sometimes even being disrespectful. We may inappropriately tell you to leave us alone, or tell an overweight person he is fat, or chastise a mother for having a noisy kid, when otherwise, we may not have spoken those obvious truths out loud. Help guard us from such social faux paus, and forgive us if we occasionally slip up.

Please ignore our grumpiness.

Likewise, a second byproduct of a stroke is the tendency to be frustrated, discouraged, and downright irritable. On those occasions, hopefully rare, please understand what we're going through, and allow us those infrequent outbursts. If it becomes a frequent occurrence, point it out to us and talk to us about it.

Do not allow us to cultivate bad habits.

If we walk with a slight limp during our recovery, there is the possibility we will allow that limp to become a part of our new normal. Please point that out. Whether a crooked smile, a restricted arm movement, or a limp, it just means we have more work to do. Feel free to point that out and encourage us to do the work. Please help us prevent newly formed bad habits from becoming a part of our new normal.

Remind us if we forget to thank you.

Most of us are eternally grateful for our caregivers, and try frequently to thank them for their kindness and giving so generously of themselves during our most vulnerable times. Occasionally, we forget. Through a loving, good-natured reminder, or some other approach, let us know if we seem ungrateful. An absence of stated appreciation is a sure fire way to foster 'caregiver burnout.' Please help us never get to that point.

Keep us focused on our ultimate goal.

Remember that our goals are normalcy and independence. In the hazy fog of our journey, it is possible that we may lose sight of those objectives. We may not remember, in the midst of our frustration, that it's not the battle, it's the war. It's a long journey. Please remind us. Remind us of the mantra from the civil rights movement, 'Keep your eyes on the prize.'

Take time for yourself.

With this new life which was suddenly thrust upon you, and the overwhelming responsibilities that go with it, your old life can potentially get lost in the shuffle. Don't allow that to happen! Take a break. Go out. Have some alone time. Meet with your friends. Find a way to get away from the burdens of taking care of us 24x7. Don't be selfish, but be sensible. Remember, you're no good to us if you're no good to yourself.

CHAPTER 12
Light at the End of the Tunnel

Day 125

HAVING SUFFERED A STROKE ON that fateful December morning, I began thinking of myself in terms of what I could and could not do. Subtly, I drifted into that mindset and the reminders were all around me. The right side of my body was paralyzed. As I progressed I still could not walk smoothly. I faced limitations with my right arm and hand. My mouth continued to droop slightly when I smiled. I went to therapy sessions three times a week. Family members and friends took care of routine, everyday tasks for me. I was chauffeured everywhere I went. My condition was apparent to others, and people went out of their way to accommodate me. Everywhere I turned, I was treated like a man with limitations.

The good news in that scenario is, I had the therapy, friends and family members there to assist me when I needed it most. The bad news is, I had begun to cultivate the mindset of a man with limitations. Subtly and almost imperceptibly, I had begun to define myself in those terms… a person of limitations!

On the occasion of my birthday, April 26, a little more than four months after my stroke, I had an epiphany. If I were going to regain my normalcy, at some point I was going to have to start thinking and acting like the man I used to be, not a man with limitations. I had to ask myself, when was I going to resume my normal life?

I decided it was time.

I still had limitations, but I concluded I would no longer allow myself to be defined in that fashion. I was going to employ the axiom, 'Fake it until you make it'. I would no longer be that person with limitations. I declared to myself and others, that from this day forward, I will be my old normal self. My physical body was still in the process of recovering. But in my mind, I declared myself recovered. I decided from this point forward, I was going to once again start doing all the things that I used to do before my stroke. I clearly could not do all those things yet, but for over four months, my stroke had become my defining characteristic. I was no longer defined as a writer, or musician, or father, or grandfather, or golfer. I was defined as someone who had suffered a stroke.

No more!

It was time to be Ross Kelly again. I decided the biggest change that needed to occur was not my ability to walk, or use my arm and hand, but my mindset. I had to remind myself to act normal again.

That was a dicey proposition to act as if I had no limitations when I obviously still did. But eventually it began to pay off. I went about doing things I had not done in months. It was not as smooth or as elegant as it once was, but I was doing them. And there were things I was still unable to do, but each day, those things became fewer.

Fake it until you make it!

One of the most joyful events following my stroke, was the rescheduled launch of the writing workshop that had been delayed. The Flowery Branch Writing Club is a group of mostly women, eager to write their stories, and they agreed to wait patiently until my recovery was sufficient to conduct the workshop. Next to writing itself, this was the type of opportunity I loved most, and the type of group I enjoyed being with. The wine and the champagne flowed and was topped off by gourmet cooking. If there is a better way to recover from a stroke, I cannot imagine what it would be.

This group was fun, serious about their writing, and full of life. They were just what I needed during a critical stretch of my recovery. Even though I was not yet fully recovered, they re-engaged me in life, doing the things I loved. That, as much as anything, was the most enjoyable and meaningful thing I had done since my stroke occurred, and I'm forever grateful for the role they played in my eventual recovery.

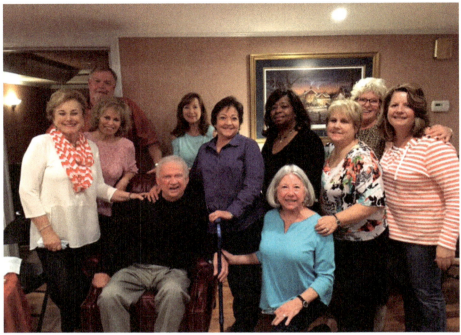

Flowery Branch Writer's Club:
L to R: Seated: Me, Robbie Harrison; Standing: Freddie Clifton Law,
Rob Horton, Linda Medders, Betty Zegar, Cheryl Thompson, Catherine
Myrick, Liz Nietzke, Ellen Montgomery, Jane Blake.

Organized by my cousin, Freddie Clifton Law, to whom I am eternally grateful, rather than being in a hospital bed or in the gymnasium undergoing therapy, she helped me reclaim my life. I was not one hundred percent yet, but the workshop re-introduced me to the notion of feeling normal again. The group had become a part of my recovery. They were able to monitor my progress from week to week, over the course of the six-week workshop, and give me feedback on what I was and was not able to do. Thank you, Freddie and the members of the Flowery Branch Writing Club. You helped me, once again, regain my normalcy.

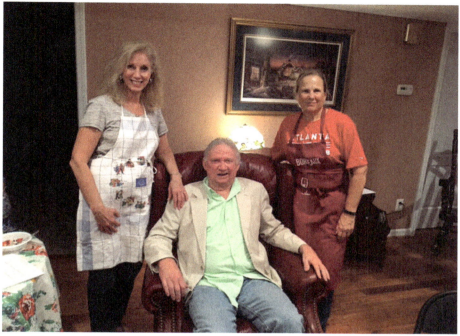

Flowery Branch Chefs: L to R: Beverly Martin, Me, Cherie Stark.

In addition to the Flowery Branch Book Club, I had other events to look forward to...

At the end of April, some four months after my stroke, I was scheduled to run in a 5K road race with my children and grandchildren. Looking ahead to that road race was a major motivator for me and would be living proof that my life had returned to normal. I realize if I participate, I will be walking the course this year, not running. But the mere notion of participating at all will be a major accomplishment.

Additionally, one of my granddaughters was getting married Memorial Day weekend, some five months post stroke. Dancing at that wedding would also be one of the most momentous occasions of my life.

I had another event, planned later for the summer, to take a family trip to the islands. That, too, would serve as a milestone event towards being back into the realm of normalcy.

I am one of four brothers. One of the joys the four of us have shared for more than 40 years are our annual golf outings. From Torrey Pines in California to Ponte Vedra in Florida, we have delighted in our golf competitions, and have every intention of continuing the tradition. The question that was obviously on everyone's mind after my stroke was, would we be able to continue?

Our next scheduled outing was scheduled for the spring of 2017, in Kitty Hawk, North Carolina, which would be a mere five or six months following my stroke. Now a stroke can easily disrupt your schedule, but I had no intention of allowing one to get in the way of our annual golf outings. Though we delayed our annual outing to the fall, we planned to resume our golf competitions, and the bets and the competition will continue to be as intense as always.

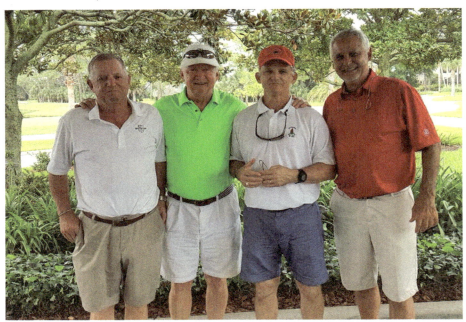

Me and my three brothers after a round, in Ponte Vedra, Florida.
From L to R, Bill, Me, Mike and Pete.

Day 140

I T HAS NOW BEEN NEARLY five months since my stroke. The road has indeed been long and winding, and the end is close but I am not yet over the finish line. My standing and walking motion, my right arm and hand motion, and my speech have regained some sense of normalcy, but I'm still cautious. I still continue to stand up from a chair in a slow and deliberate manner, and I continue to look straight ahead and concentrate fully when I walk, refusing to look around for fear of being distracted and losing my balance. And I continue to occasionally use my left hand instead of my once damaged right. But after five months, I am once again living life.

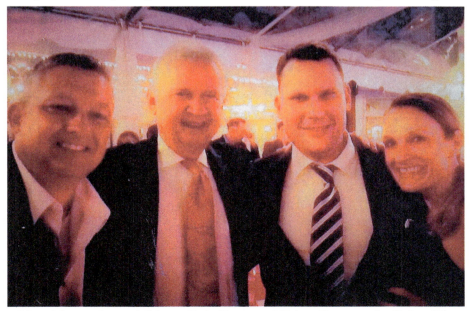

Me with my three children: Rob, Brett and Erin. Once again, living life.

There are many habits that I cultivated during my recovery which persist today. Some are good and some not so good. Those habits are now a part of the new and improved me, and my new normal.

When will all this end? When will I resume being normal"?

"It all depends. Every situation is different."

I have come to accept the response to those questions that the medical professionals had told me from the very beginning. Perhaps the answer is, maybe never. Maybe I'll simply continue a journey that does not reach a destination, but is a road of continuous improvement. Perhaps that is the journey. Perhaps the journey never ends.

Maybe that is the normal that resided within me all along, and it took a stroke to discover it.

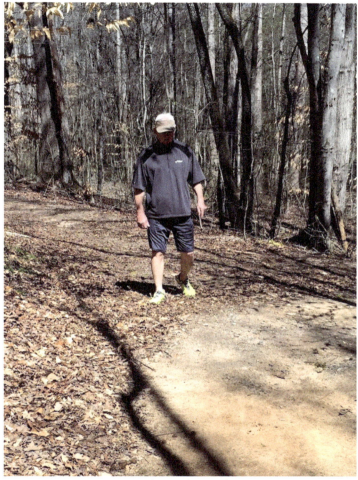

Back on the trail.

Maybe my new normal is continuing to live my life to the fullest, but with a new and improved perspective!

EPILOGUE

WHEN I BEGAN WRITING THIS book, my premise was, 'It's all about the work.' Some six months later, I still believe that to be true. It's about doing the work and having the right attitude. I thought that combination would be the key to a successful recovery. Attitude, as much as work, appeared to be essential to success. I recall the 90 something year-old working in the therapy room, willingly and joyfully, and dedicated to his recovery, as opposed to the man half his age begrudgingly doing only what was asked of him. The right attitude, it seemed, was as essential as the work itself.

Okay, so it's work and the right attitude.

But when something like this happens, the tendency is to fight it. When we have illnesses, we fight. That is the natural inclination. That is what we are taught to do. We fight with all of our might to prevent the illness from winning. The last thing we think about is giving into it. But what about when your body needs your permission to heal itself? That is what the body needs when recovering from a stroke. Maybe that is the key… to give in to it. Let the body takeover.

So maybe it's about doing the work, having the right attitude and the willingness to give in to a journey that is not of your choosing. Maybe that's the right combination.

But, oh those lonely nights, thinking and wondering when does it all happen? When will it all be over? And being told when I endlessly asked, 'It depends. Every situation is different.' How many times was I told I have to be patient? How many times was I told that patience would be the key to this journey?

Okay, so work, the right attitude, give in to it, and patience.

But again, I was constantly reminded, the body can do its work only when it's had plenty of rest. Rest, something I was neither familiar with nor good at, was a critical factor, I was told. I remember those endless nights at 3 AM when I was supposed to be sleeping, but was exercising instead. I had to frequently be reminded that rest would be critical to my recovery.

Okay, I've got it. It's the work, the right attitude, give in to it, patience, and plenty of rest.

But how did I sustain myself through this grueling and frustrating journey? Who did I turn to in my loneliest, most frustrating moments? During those same nights at 3 AM, when the nurses had finished their duties, and it was just me alone with my thoughts, the presence of God was there with me. None of the other components, the work, the attitude, patience, and rest, would have been possible had I not had my ultimate faith in God. I cannot count the number of occasions when during my most frustrating moments, I had to seek assurance from God that I would achieve some form of recovery. And miraculously, each time I sought that assurance, it was there, and I carried on.

Maybe *that* was the formula. Work, a good attitude, give in to it, patience, plenty of rest, all working together with a solid faith as the foundation.

Then I was reminded that I could not have achieved any of this without a proper support group. I was reminded of the endless visits of my family and friends. I was reminded of those who acted as caregivers, who cooked my meals, did my laundry, took out my trash, and the many other functions that I once took for granted but could no longer perform. How could I have achieved my recovery without those individuals so lovingly giving of themselves?

Okay, so now I had my formula … My faith in God that the work would ultimately pay off, accompanied by the right attitude, giving in to it patience, plenty of rest, and a caring support group.

But in the end, I realized, none of those other things mattered if I was not willing to do the work. They were all part and parcel of doing the work.

So it *does* all come down to doing the work!

There is an expression that says, 'The instructions only make sense after the bicycle has been put together.' That was certainly true in my case. It was only after having endured the endless days and nights of doing the work and wondering when I would see the results, that I began to understand what was truly required of me. It was only then that I understood what I would have to do if this were to ever happen again.

But that would be for someone else's benefit, not mine. I was highly sensitive to the possibility of a second or third stroke, but I had no intentions of going through this experience again, no matter how wonderful the medical staff, or the friends, or the family… and no matter how special or meaningful the fraternity of which I was now a part.

A second stroke was not in my plans. I had too much to accomplish, and too many places to go. I was too determined, too active, too young and far too healthy for such a debilitating injury again.

In the midst of the process, after learning I could achieve a full recovery, I was reminded very poignantly by my daughter and sister-in-law, "What have you lost?" You've had four months to re-learn how to walk, how to talk and how to use your arm. And you have a new topic to write about that will benefit others, based on first-hand experience. And in the process, you took a break from the rat race.

In reality, they were right.

What had I lost?

In many ways, I realize my journey may not have been the journey of other stroke survivors. As the doctors and therapists continued to tell me, 'Every situation is different.' I had wonderful healthcare, a foundation of good health, and a wonderful family and group of friends. Without the benefit of any of those, I would possibly not have recovered, or be able to write this book, or even be here today. But I believe the choices and the potential outcomes remain the same: death, debilitation, or a full recovery. Which do you choose?

I do realize the state of one's health and the severity of the stroke may determine the first outcome. Death is a reality that is far too common with strokes. But it is not inevitable. Health and lifestyle choices should be made before a stroke occurs, not after. Though there are many factors beyond our control, such as age, race, and family history, many other choices remain within our control.

Debilitation or some form of recurring effect from a stroke is also a choice. Assuming one has survived the first outcome, the second outcome is dependent mostly on the individual. Do I want to walk with a recurring limp or do I want to walk as I did before? Do I want to talk with a slur or do I want to talk as I did before? Do I want to live with limited use of my hand and shoulder, or do I want the movement I enjoyed before? The answer to all of these questions mostly comes down to one more question: How hard am I willing to work to achieve my pre-stroke normalcy?

I was heartened to learn the answer... 'As long and as hard as it takes.'

That is the fraternity of which I am now proud to be associated. That is the fraternity that will help eventually eliminate or dramatically diminish this health scourge that haunts so many of us. I never chose to join this fraternity, but now that I am in it, I am prepared to do my part to reduce it in size, and make it a little more difficult to join.

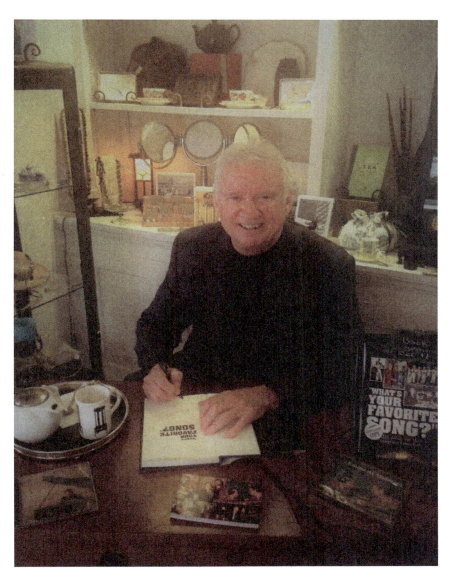

Ross has resumed his writing career and speaking engagements, and is available to tell his story. To book him as a speaker for your upcoming event or to arrange a writing workshop in your area, please contact him at rosskelly426@gmail.com.

CPSIA information can be obtained
at www.ICGtesting.com
Printed in the USA
LVOW06*2020280917

550474LV00027B/160/P